TAKE CONTROL
OF YOUR
PREDIABETES
AND
TYPE 2 DIABETES

TAKE CONTROL OF YOUR PREDIABETES AND TYPE 2 DIABETES

Prevent, manage and reverse your condition

Dr Val Wilson

GREEN TREE
LONDON · OXFORD · NEW YORK · NEW DELHI · SYDNEY

GREEN TREE
Bloomsbury Publishing Plc
50 Bedford Square, London, WC1B 3DP, UK
Bloomsbury Publishing Ireland Limited,
29 Earlsfort Terrace, Dublin 2, D02 AY28, Ireland

BLOOMSBURY, GREEN TREE and the Green Tree logo are trademarks of
Bloomsbury Publishing Plc

First published in Great Britain 2026

Copyright © Dr Val Wilson, 2026

Dr Val Wilson has asserted her right under the Copyright, Designs and Patents Act,
1988, to be identified as Author of this work

For legal purposes the Acknowledgements on p. 198 constitute
an extension of this copyright page

All rights reserved. No part of this publication may be: i) reproduced or transmitted in any form, electronic or mechanical, including photocopying, recording or by means of any information storage or retrieval system without prior permission in writing from the publishers; or ii) used or reproduced in any way for the training, development or operation of artificial intelligence (AI) technologies, including generative AI technologies. The rights holders expressly reserve this publication from the text and data mining exception as per Article 4(3) of the Digital Single Market Directive (EU) 2019/790

Bloomsbury Publishing Plc does not have any control over, or responsibility for, any third-party websites referred to or in this book. All internet addresses given in this book were correct at the time of going to press. The author and publisher regret any inconvenience caused if addresses have changed or sites have ceased to exist, but can accept no responsibility for any such changes

Disclaimer: The material contained in this book is for informational purposes only. No material in this publication is intended to be a substitute for professional medical advice, diagnosis or treatment. Always seek the advice of your GP or other qualified health care professional with any questions you may have regarding a medical condition, including mental health concerns, or treatment and before undertaking a new healthcare regime, and never disregard professional medical advice or delay in seeking it because of something you have read in this book

All case studies in this book are based on real experiences, but names and identifying details have been changed to protect the privacy of individuals

A catalogue record for this book is available from the British Library

Library of Congress Cataloguing-in-Publication data has been applied for

ISBN: TPB: 978-1-3994-2375-5; eBook: 978-1-3994-2373-1

2 4 6 8 10 9 7 5 3 1

Typeset in Ballinger by Lumina Datamatics Ltd
Printed and bound in Great Britain by Clays Ltd, Elcograf S.p.A.

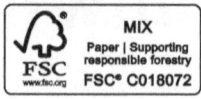

To find out more about our authors and books visit www.bloomsbury.com
and sign up for our newsletters

For product safety related questions contact productsafety@bloomsbury.com

For Neil

Contents

Introduction 9
    What exactly is diabetes? 10
    How to use this book 12
    About me 12

Part I: Understanding prediabetes and diabetes 15

1. **Exploring definitions of diabetes** 16
    What is prediabetes? 17
    What is type 2 diabetes? 18
2. **Physical symptoms of diabetes** 21
    What are the key symptoms? 22
    What to do if you spot symptoms 24
3. **Risk factors you can control** 26
    Why it is important to control risk 27
    The lifestyle factors you can change 29
4. **Risk factors you can't control** 40
    Fixed risk factors 40
    Am I at high risk? 42
5. **Chronic complications** 55
    What to look out for 56
    Close-up on long-term issues 57
    Other warning signs 70

Part II: Actioning change 73

6. Mindset changes 74
Beginning the process of change 75
Embracing the challenge 93

7. Physical changes 96
Weight loss through diet and exercise 97
Reducing blood glucose levels 121
Lowering blood pressure and blood cholesterol 142
Stopping smoking 147
Going to medical appointments 150

8. Emotional health 155
Responding to a diagnosis 156
Managing diabetes 162
Improving your emotional health 165

A final note 170 • **Glossary** 171 • **Resources** 177
References 181 • **Acknowledgements** 198 • **Index** 199

Introduction

If you're worried about getting diabetes, or if you already have it, then believe me you're not alone. According to Diabetes UK, in 2024 12.1 million adults in the UK were living with either diabetes or **prediabetes**. In the US, which has a population nearly five times that of the UK, 2021 data suggests 38.4 million adults have type 2 diabetes and 97.6 million have prediabetes. These are serious numbers and they highlight a serious issue, because if diabetes remains undetected or untreated for years, or even several months, it can lead to health problems, such as changes to the heart and circulatory system, eyes, kidneys, nervous system and digestive system. Of course, I understand that this might sound rather daunting, but I've written this book to reassure you and to help you to:

- Reduce your risk of developing prediabetes in the future
- Understand your prediabetes diagnosis and prevent or delay the development of type 2 diabetes for as long as possible
- Improve or reverse your type 2 diabetes if you already have it.

Take Control of Your Prediabetes and Type 2 Diabetes puts you firmly in charge of your future health. It gives you the information you need to make informed decisions and it guides you through all the lifestyle changes you can make to prevent and manage your condition, including supporting positive mental health (*see* chapter 8). In the following chapters I'll explain in detail what diabetes is and how to deal with it, but let's begin with a short overview – and for that you'll need to know three key terms:

- **Glucose**: Also known as 'blood sugar' when it's present in your bloodstream, glucose is a type of sugar that's found in lots of different foods and is a primary source of energy for the cells in your body. In this book I talk a lot about 'blood glucose levels'.

- **Insulin**: A hormone produced by your pancreas, insulin plays a crucial role in regulating your blood glucose levels, allowing the cells in your body to take up glucose from your bloodstream, so that those cells can either use the glucose for energy now or store it to use later.
- **Insulin resistance**: If the cells in your body don't respond to insulin and don't take up the glucose in your bloodstream, the condition is called *insulin resistance*. This leads to a build-up of glucose, raising your blood glucose levels, and increases your risk of prediabetes and type 2 diabetes.

What exactly is diabetes?

If you're a healthy person the amount of glucose in your blood is constantly changing. It rises when you consume food containing glucose and falls when your body uses the glucose to fuel metabolic functions such as heartbeat, brain activity and movement. Insulin's role is to allow the glucose in your blood to be taken up by your cells, enabling the energy it delivers to be either used immediately or stored for later. However, when your body becomes insulin resistant the glucose isn't absorbed into your cells and builds up in your blood instead. High blood glucose levels are the key feature of prediabetes and type 2 diabetes, and over time high levels of glucose in your blood cause damage to your cells and other organs, and you are likely to face significant health problems.

There are a number of factors that put you at risk of developing prediabetes and type 2 diabetes, but one of the most significant is having too much fat stored around your liver and pancreas. This is what's known as visceral fat and, although it's more common in people who are overweight, those who are a healthy weight can have it, too. The science is quite complex, but visceral fat seems to disrupt the way insulin works, leading to that build-up of glucose in the bloodstream, and ultimately the development of prediabetes and type 2 diabetes.

The great news, though, is that with lifestyle changes involving healthy eating, increased physical activity and weight loss, you can lower high blood glucose levels and help prevent, delay or reverse prediabetes or type 2 diabetes by enabling your body to use insulin more effectively.

FREQUENTLY ASKED QUESTIONS

Let's look at some of the most common questions people have about diabetes.

Can prediabetes and type 2 diabetes be cured or reversed?
Yes! Most people can cure or reverse prediabetes and type 2 diabetes if they make changes to their lifestyle, unless those conditions have occurred due to old age, ethnicity, genetics or certain medications (for more on this, see chapter 4).

Can you manage prediabetes and type 2 diabetes?
Yes! Whatever your diabetes status – undiagnosed or diagnosed with prediabetes or type 2 diabetes – with the right lifestyle changes (as outlined in this book), you can manage your condition to live a longer, healthier life (for more on this, see chapter 3).

Can you explain the different types of diabetes?
Yes, of course! Prediabetes means your blood glucose levels (blood sugar) are higher than normal, but not high enough for you to be diagnosed with type 2 diabetes. If you do receive a type 2 diagnosis, it will be because your body can no longer use or produce insulin effectively – you have become insulin resistant.

Type 1 diabetes, on the other hand, is an autoimmune disease in which your body is unable to produce insulin, because your immune system repeatedly destroys insulin-producing cells in your pancreas. Only 8% of people with diabetes have type 1, although you can develop it at any age, but it is often diagnosed in childhood. It is treated by taking insulin, but there is no cure and it can't be reversed by lifestyle changes. These factors make type 1 diabetes very different from prediabetes and type 2, so this book doesn't focus on type 1.

As you read this, perhaps you have already been diagnosed with prediabetes or type 2 diabetes. Or perhaps you haven't been diagnosed yet, but you may know that there is type 2 diabetes in your family, or think you may develop it because type 2 diabetes is a possible side effect of your prescribed medication. However, if this is you, please don't worry, because although everyone's situation and health status is different, in many cases these conditions can be reversed and in all cases they can be vastly improved.

> **FACT: If you currently have prediabetes, you can act now to stop type 2 diabetes developing at a later date. Having full-blown type 2 diabetes is also a lot harder to live with than prediabetes, so it's worth doing the work to prevent it.**

How to use this book

The book is divided into two parts. I think it really helps if you have a basic understanding of the effect of glucose and insulin on your body, so Part I is designed to be informative. I look at definitions, symptoms, risk factors and some of the complications that can occur if diabetes is left unaddressed. Part II, on the other hand, focuses on the changes you need to make to your lifestyle to manage, improve or reverse prediabetes and type 2 diabetes, and suggests strategies to help you do that. Everything you need to know is covered (important words appear in bold italics and are featured in the glossary – see pp. 171–6) and I have included lots of facts and tips. I have also used real-life stories in each chapter to show how other people have dealt with some of the issues that you may be facing. Most of what I have to say applies to both prediabetes and type 2 diabetes, and if you're new to these conditions it makes sense to read Part I first, but it's not essential, so feel free to go straight to Part II if you're ready to start making changes to your lifestyle now.

About me

Before we get started, you may wonder what qualifies me to write this book. Well, I have been an academic for over 30 years and have a Doctorate in Diabetes Health Education. My mission is to inform, educate and support others with diabetes to achieve a good quality of life, and, as a specialist in this field, I have advised the UK government and NHS on diabetes strategies, and conducted many studies looking at how and why people self-manage their diabetes. I have also carried out more than 10 years of voluntary work with a diabetes charity and published widely on all aspects of living with, and caring for people with, diabetes. I also have diabetes myself. It's type 1 diabetes, which I've had for 50 years, and it's very unpredictable, and difficult to control and manage. However, although this book is about prediabetes and type 2 diabetes, not the type 1 that I have, I understand dealing with diabetes is daunting, but I also know that with the right strategies and approach, you really can prevent it, manage it and even reverse it over time.

Part I

Understanding prediabetes and diabetes

Chapter 1
Exploring definitions of diabetes

> This chapter looks at what prediabetes is, the various subtypes of type 2 diabetes (there are several) and how they are all diagnosed.

To do anything, including breathing and thinking, we need energy and we get that energy from a sugar called glucose. This comes from the food we eat, primarily from carbohydrates, but in order to use it as energy (or store it for later), the cells in your body need to absorb the glucose. However, they can't do that without the help of insulin, the hormone which you produce in your pancreas.

When everything is working normally, when the level of glucose in your blood rises your pancreas releases insulin, which allows the glucose to enter your cells, thus lowering the level of glucose in your blood. Then, when the level of glucose in your blood is low, the level of insulin decreases, allowing your body to release stored glucose. However, when there is not enough insulin available to deal with the amount of glucose present in your blood, or the insulin released cannot work properly, prediabetes and diabetes occur.

What is prediabetes?

You may not have heard of prediabetes, so what exactly is it? When your blood glucose levels rise above certain limits (for more on why this happens, see chapters 3 and 4), your pancreas makes extra insulin to get your body cells to respond and absorb more glucose. For a time, this extra insulin makes up for the weak response and the levels of glucose in your blood remain normal. However, your pancreas can't keep on overproducing insulin. Your blood glucose levels begin to increase and they stay raised, with the excess glucose remaining in your blood instead of entering your cells. Your blood glucose levels continue to increase and at this stage a blood test will show you have prediabetes. It may take several years, but without lifestyle changes or treatment (see Part II), type 2 diabetes then develops.

> **ALI SAYS:** *It was a real shock to be told my prediabetes has progressed so I now have type 2 diabetes. I didn't even feel ill and my prediabetes was only found because of a routine blood test.*

Prediabetes is diagnosed using several methods to measure glucose levels at different points in time. This is done to ensure that your test does not show a one-off high glucose level, which can occur due to stress, infection or illness. A **fasting plasma glucose test**, which measures the amount of glucose in the blood after fasting overnight for between eight and 12 hours, is the quickest way to determine prediabetes; an **oral glucose tolerance test** (taken by mouth) measures how well your body can produce insulin after eating a certain amount of glucose; and an **HbA1c blood test** measures the amount of glucose sticking to your red blood cells over the two- to three-month lifespan of a cell.

It is possible to have prediabetes for years without major symptoms (for more on this, see chapter 2), but high blood glucose levels cause damage over time, even though this may only become apparent when more serious health problems, such as eye, kidney or nerve disease, occur. The only way to confirm that you have elevated blood glucose levels is if your doctor arranges a blood test to measure glucose tolerance. This will show either:

- A blood glucose level less than 7.8 mmol/L (140 mg/dL in the US, because it uses different units of measurement), which is normal.
- A result between 7.8 mmol/L and 11.0 mmol/L (140 and 199 mg/dL in the US) showing that you have prediabetes.
- A reading of more than 11.1 mmol/L (200 mg/dL in the US) two hours after eating, showing that you have type 2 diabetes.

Being diagnosed with prediabetes is a warning sign that your body is not dealing with glucose very well. If you don't make changes to your lifestyle, your risk of type 2 diabetes will increase. If you begin to lose weight (this means losing 5% of your body weight) and exercise more (moderate and regular exercise means 30 minutes of activity, such as brisk walking, five days a week), your risk will go down considerably. If you already have type 2, many people can reverse this with lifestyle changes.

> **FACT: Being diagnosed with prediabetes is a warning sign that type 2 diabetes is ahead. If you continue along the same road your risk of type 2 diabetes will increase. Not everyone with prediabetes goes on to develop full-blown type 2 diabetes, but over three to five years around 25% of people will.**

What is type 2 diabetes?

Prediabetes doesn't occur ahead of a type 1 diabetes diagnosis. Type 1 is an auto-immune condition that cannot be reversed and treatment involves managing your blood glucose levels by taking insulin every day. What's more, it only makes up 8% of diabetes cases, which is why this book doesn't focus on this condition. Type 2, however, makes up

90–95% of cases and is a chronic metabolic condition in which your body becomes resistant to the hormone insulin. This means insulin isn't able to facilitate the absorption of glucose into your cells, leading to high levels of glucose in your blood.

Type 2 diabetes is usually diagnosed in people who are over 40 years of age, but due to inactive lifestyles and diets high in refined carbohydrates it is now increasingly seen in children and young people. In fact, we are currently in the midst of a diabetes epidemic. It's estimated that 415 million people globally – or one in 11 of the world's adult population – are living with diabetes, although almost half of all global type 2 diabetes cases remain undiagnosed, because there are no specific symptoms. This means that any secondary health problems (see chapter 5) resulting from prolonged high glucose levels also go undiagnosed.

> **PAUL SAYS:** *At first when my doctor confirmed I had type 2 diabetes I found it hard to accept, because I'm only 33, but once the news had sunk in, I was able to start looking at my lifestyle choices.*

If you are diagnosed with type 2 diabetes – and the test for high glucose levels is the same as for prediabetes – it can be managed with lifestyle modifications, such as dietary changes and increasing physical activity levels, and/or by taking diabetes medicines by mouth. However, sometimes these methods fail to reduce blood glucose levels over time and insulin may be prescribed.

> **FACT:** Insulin resistance is when your cells become less sensitive to insulin or don't respond to it, so the insulin isn't able to do its job of regulating glucose properly, causing glucose levels in your blood to increase. If those glucose levels become high enough, it causes type 2 diabetes. However, for people with insulin resistance

and prediabetes, physical activity, a healthy diet and weight loss can reduce diabetes risk by 58%.

✳ Key messages ✳

- Prediabetes is when your blood glucose levels rise above certain limits, because not all the insulin produced by your pancreas is able to work correctly.

- If your blood glucose levels continue to rise, you are likely to develop type 2 diabetes.

- This book focuses on prediabetes and type 2 diabetes.

Chapter 2
Physical symptoms of diabetes

> This chapter helps you spot the symptoms of diabetes quickly, so you can report them to your doctor as early as possible. This is important because the symptoms can easily go undetected.

Both prediabetes and type 2 diabetes have the same symptoms, because both are caused by elevated glucose levels, but those symptoms can be hard to recognise, which is why it's particularly important to be aware of what they are.

Symptoms can be very general, like feeling constantly tired, which means they can easily be put down to having a busy life, or you simply may not notice them. For instance, you may not register that your cuts and bruises are slow to heal or assume you feel thirstier or need to urinate more often because you're getting old. However, even if you experience mild changes in your health, it is important to tell your doctor about them.

If prediabetes continues untreated, then it can eventually develop into type 2 diabetes. If symptoms of high blood glucose levels in type 2 diabetes are ignored then chronic complications – secondary health problems caused by high blood glucose levels – can eventually occur and may affect your eyesight, heart, kidneys and nerves.

What are the key symptoms?

There are nine main day-to-day symptoms associated with high blood glucose levels:

1. **Needing to urinate more often**: You might notice that you have to get up several times during the night, which is prompted by your body's attempt to rid itself of excess glucose by producing more urine.

2. **Often feeling thirsty**: The trouble is, having a drink doesn't quench your thirst, because you become dehydrated when there is excess glucose, which your body tries to eliminate, so you drink more and urinate more to flush it out.

3. **Feeling tired most of the time**: If day-to-day activities are an effort it's because your body cells are unable to process the glucose needed for energy.

4. **Weight loss**: Obviously if you have been dieting or more active than usual then there is a reason for your weight loss, but if you're losing weight without a good reason, this can be because your body's cells are starved of the fuel they need and cannot use the excess glucose in the blood without adequate insulin.

5. **Blurred vision**: This is due to excess glucose causing swelling, including in the lenses of your eyes, and other general changes to your eyes.

6. **Itching**: You may notice itchiness around the genitals in particular. Thrush infections can also occur due to high levels of glucose in the blood and urine.

7. **Cuts, scratches and bruises**: These may take weeks or months to heal as a result of high blood glucose and poor circulation.

8. **Tingling or numbness**: If you get this kind of sensation in your hands, feet or toes it could be because of nerve damage.

9. **Darker skin**: This might appear in the armpits or sides of the neck, and you might get small skin growths or skin tags, all due to high blood glucose levels.

Just a reminder: prediabetes describes blood glucose levels that are higher than normal, but not yet high enough to be diagnosed as full-blown type 2 diabetes. However, even if prediabetes develops into undiagnosed type 2 diabetes, the symptoms tend to be mild, so they are not always obvious, meaning small changes can go unreported. However, high blood glucose levels can affect all the systems in your body, which is why it is so important to get any symptoms of high glucose checked and treated before permanent damage can occur and complications are triggered (for more on complications, *see* chapter 5).

TAHMIDA SAYS: *I feel a bit embarrassed saying this, but I thought that glucose was a good thing in the body as it gives you energy, so the more you have, the better it is. I used to have energy drinks every day, which are pure glucose and caffeine, because my energy was often flagging at work. I was tired when I got up and by mid-morning I felt exhausted. I used to sit in my car at lunchtime to have a snooze. The energy drinks obviously didn't help and made things worse. A friend noticed this and pointed out that I might have diabetes, because I was also always drinking coffee, but still felt tired. She was right. Some blood tests showed a high glucose result – my body hadn't been able to process all that glucose I was consuming. I got some proper advice, stopped the energy drinks and made changes to my diet. I feel so much better now!*

SHOULD I SEE MY DOCTOR?

The symptoms of high glucose levels, and thus prediabetes and type 2 diabetes, are not always clear-cut, which is why it's important to find out whether you have a higher risk of developing these conditions (see chapter 3). However, the three main changes you may notice, and which you should report to your doctor, are:

1. Frequently feeling thirsty, even though you've had something to drink.

2. Having to urinate more often, especially during the night, because you are drinking more.

3. Feeling tired all the time over a period of weeks or months.

What to do if you spot symptoms

If you suspect that you may have prediabetes or type 2 diabetes, visit your doctor as soon as possible to get a proper diagnosis and discuss suitable management options. Be prepared to discuss any of the symptoms you are experiencing, such as itching, increased thirst, frequent urination, unexplained weight loss, feeling tired, slow wound healing or blurred vision. Your doctor will suggest you have a blood test to check your blood glucose levels. A specific blood test, called an HbA1c test, is usually used to determine the amount of glucose present in red blood cells over the previous three months, but a fasting plasma glucose test or an oral glucose tolerance test might also be used (see chapter 1). Based on the results of your test, your doctor will explain the diagnosis and discuss the next steps.

Over the short term – three to five years – only about 25% of people with prediabetes go on to develop type 2 diabetes. Diabetes UK estimates that with the right support, up to 50% of people with prediabetes can prevent or delay type 2 diabetes. This is why it's important to recognise potential symptoms early and report them quickly.

FACT: If you're looking on the internet for information about increased blood glucose levels, this condition is also known medically as:

- ***Impaired fasting glucose*** (IFG)
- Impaired glucose regulation (IGR)
- ***Impaired glucose tolerance*** (IGT)
- Non-diabetic ***hyperglycaemia***

Once a blood sample has been taken to detect high glucose levels your doctor will arrange a laboratory blood test, such as the HbA1c test, which shows your average blood glucose level over the past three months. An alternative to this is a fasting glucose test, which measures your blood glucose level after not eating or drinking anything but water for eight hours. A glucose tolerance test is also used, where, after a fasting blood test, you are given a glucose drink, followed by a second test two hours later to measure the amount of glucose in your blood. These laboratory blood tests are used to make an official diagnosis of prediabetes or type 2 diabetes.

✳ Key messages ✳

- Both prediabetes and type 2 diabetes have the same symptoms, because they are both caused by elevated glucose levels.

- Symptoms can be very general, like feeling constantly tired, which is easily ignored, or dismissed as due to something else, such as having a busy life.

- Prediabetes may remain invisible until it develops into type 2 diabetes, but even at this stage many people don't experience any specific symptoms of the condition.

- Even if you have mild changes in your health, it is important that you tell your doctor.

Chapter 3

Risk factors you can control

This chapter prepares you to take charge of your own diabetes health by describing what will increase your chances of developing prediabetes or type 2 diabetes – or of already having one of these conditions.

It is important to understand the potential risks associated with developing prediabetes or type 2 diabetes that you can control, because this will help you make informed decisions and take appropriate preventative measures. Lifestyle factors such as eating a high-calorie and high-fat diet, taking little or no exercise, smoking, poor sleep and even where you live can make it more likely that you will develop diabetes. However, most people can stop the onset of prediabetes and type 2 diabetes by making changes to their diet and exercise routines (for more on how to do this, *see* Part II). You may not know you have prediabetes or even full-blown diabetes, though, so if you have one or more of the risk factors discussed in this chapter, particularly if you are overweight or a close family member has or had type 2 diabetes, you should be tested.

> **FACT: Recognising your risk is the first step to prevention as there are a number of steps you can take to tackle the onset of prediabetes and type 2 diabetes.**

Why it is important to control risk

Reducing your risk of developing prediabetes and type 2 diabetes may be something you have never considered, especially if you feel fit and healthy right now. However, don't be fooled into thinking that the 'pre' gives you plenty of time to consider possible lifestyle changes or that prediabetes doesn't pose a significant threat to your health. You can have prediabetes for years without experiencing any symptoms, which means you won't know there is anything wrong until you are affected by serious health problems. The great news, though, is that prediabetes, and potentially even type 2 diabetes, is reversible.

> **FACT: One in 10 adults now risk developing type 2 diabetes by the year 2035, but walking for 15 minutes after meals could prevent type 2 diabetes.**

You may currently have diagnosed or undiagnosed prediabetes, but you also need to be aware that you are at risk of developing type 2 diabetes in the future. Research has shown that making certain changes to your lifestyle, such as eating more healthily and increasing the amount of physical activity you do, both of which will help you lose weight, can reduce your risk of developing type 2 diabetes by 50%.

That's important because type 2 diabetes has multiple risk factors and delayed diagnosis allows damage to your cells due to elevated blood glucose levels to worsen over time. This cell damage can ultimately cause a range of serious secondary health conditions, such as sight problems, impaired kidney function, heart and blood vessel disease, stroke and nerve damage. These are known as chronic complications (see chapter 5) and they occur because in the long run ongoing high blood glucose levels damage structures in your body.

> ## WHEN AGE MEANS LIFESTYLE CHANGES WON'T WORK
>
> Type 2 diabetes usually occurs in those who are over the age of 40 due to lifestyle issues, but some older people in their seventies or eighties may not be able to produce adequate amounts of insulin when they eat, due to the ageing of the insulin-producing cells in their pancreas, so the concentration of glucose in their blood rises to above normal levels. This means that lifestyle factors are not the reason for their prediabetes and type 2 diabetes, but it also means that they can't reverse this condition with healthy eating, more exercise and weight loss (see chapter 4). There isn't a specific age at which someone can no longer reverse type 2 diabetes, but the longer you've had the condition, the more challenging the reversal becomes.

Prediabetes and type 2 diabetes share almost all the same risk factors for long-term health problems, but if you already have prediabetes, this is an added risk factor as it makes you more likely to eventually develop type 2 diabetes. However, while having an increased risk of type 2 diabetes doesn't necessarily mean you will go on to develop the condition, it is still sensible to make some lifestyle changes to reduce the risk as much as possible. Invisible changes occur in the body when blood glucose levels are higher than they should be, and over time this does damage to the cell structures of organs and tissues, altering their ability to function. This can only be confirmed by an HbA1c blood test to detect prolonged high blood glucose levels.

In many cases it is possible to prevent or delay prediabetes and type 2 diabetes by making simple changes to your diet to reduce your bodyweight and by increasing the amount of exercise you do (for more on how to make sustainable dietary and exercise changes, see Part II).

If you are at risk of prediabetes or type 2 diabetes, your doctor will help you find out what will work best for you.

The lifestyle factors you can change

In the UK, 13.6 million people are currently at increased risk of developing type 2 diabetes – and a diagnosis of prediabetes acts as a real wake-up call, a warning that you need to take action to reduce your risk of developing full-blown type 2 diabetes. However, it also means that there is the perfect opportunity for prevention and fortunately, there are several areas where you can reduce your risk of prediabetes and type 2 diabetes:

1. Weight loss and exercise
2. Sleep
3. Smoking
4. Metabolic syndrome
5. High blood glucose levels
6. High blood pressure
7. Where you live

Weight loss and exercise

You're at risk of both prediabetes and type 2 diabetes if you:

- Are overweight or have obesity
- Are physically active less than three times a week.

Research shows that for those at high risk of developing type 2, losing weight can reduce this risk by as much as 58%, while regular exercise reduces the risk by 64%. With lifestyle changes and support the chance of prediabetes developing into type 2 diabetes can be reduced or delayed by 50%.

> **LINDA SAYS:** *When my doctor told me I had prediabetes, I was completely confused. My first reaction was to ask if this meant that I did now have diabetes or if it meant I wasn't going to get it. I don't have diabetes at the moment – it was confirmed – but there's a high chance of me getting it in future if I don't change my lifestyle.*

Remember that there are several lifestyle issues that you can change to substantially reduce your risk of developing type 2 diabetes, the two main ones being maintaining a healthy weight and taking more exercise. Remember that obesity makes it hard for your body to sustain healthy blood glucose levels, while fat deposits around the waist increase your risk of insulin not working properly – insulin resistance.

> **KERRY SAYS:** *To be honest, there were several reasons why I suddenly decided to reduce my diabetes risk. My grandmother died from type 2 diabetes six months ago, so I am determined not to end up like her. I was fed up with feeling fat and breathless when I tried to do anything, like carrying laundry upstairs or pushing a lawnmower around the garden. I decided that if I cared about myself, I should do something about it. I started eating proper meals with vegetables or brown rice – small but effective food swaps instead of chips with everything. I also started walking every day, either to the shops or library, or just around the local park. Now I look forward to my healthier meals and my walks. I've lost weight over the last six months, although I don't know how much because I didn't weigh myself before I started, but now I feel more comfortable in my clothes, have more energy and I'm no longer breathless.*

Exercise is crucial for reducing the risk of prediabetes and type 2 diabetes, because it improves the sensitivity of the cells in your body to insulin and helps your blood glucose levels. Regular physical activity helps the body use insulin more effectively, which prevents the build-up of glucose in the blood. Additionally, exercise can help with weight management, which is a significant factor in the development of type 2 diabetes.

Sleep

Getting the right amount of sleep is vital for health and wellbeing. There is overwhelming evidence that, probably due to hormonal and nervous system variations, getting less than six hours' sleep a night makes you four and a half times more likely to have high levels of blood glucose, increasing your risk of prediabetes and type 2 diabetes.

Multiple studies have shown that waking repeatedly during the night, not getting enough sleep or sleeping for too long, and irregular sleep patterns all encourage glucose intolerance and insulin resistance. Furthermore, if a person already has prediabetes or type 2 diabetes, poor sleep will worsen the condition, increasing insulin resistance and blood glucose levels.

Even partial sleep deprivation over one night increases insulin resistance, which can in turn increase blood glucose levels, and having prolonged periods of poor sleep increases the risk of prediabetes progressing to type 2 diabetes.

If a period of seven to eight hours' sleep is disturbed or your patterns of sleep alter for a period of time, such as during shift work or with a new baby, you will have insulin resistance. This means that your body cells don't respond well to insulin, so it is less efficient at reducing elevated blood glucose levels and more insulin is then produced in response.

Insulin resistance is another risk factor for type 2 diabetes and people who sleep during the day and work at night often develop this condition, because shift work causes the hormone **melatonin**, which regulates waking and sleeping, to be released at the wrong times. All hormones have an impact on one another and melatonin stops insulin working effectively, causing elevated blood glucose levels in response to eating food during the night.

People with prediabetes or type 2 diabetes often have sleep problems due to unstable blood glucose levels and having to get up frequently to urinate, because their kidneys produce more urine in an attempt to flush out the excess glucose. High blood glucose during the night can lead to an inability to sleep (**insomnia**) and feeling tired the following day. Having a high blood glucose level may also cause headaches, increased thirst and tiredness that can interfere with falling asleep.

BUSHRA SAYS: *I've always had difficulty sleeping and eventually I developed prediabetes, although I didn't know the two were linked. My doctor prescribed sleeping pills about a year ago, telling me I needed a good seven hours of solid sleep each night to help reverse insulin resistance. I stopped drinking caffeinated coffee and alcohol, which helped a bit, too. The best thing has been a change in bedtime routine. I used to be on my laptop or phone late in the evenings. Now I have a bath to relax me and then always get to bed by 10.30 each night. This has definitely made a difference. I'm sleeping an average of six hours a night and my doctor says my glucose levels have now come down to near normal. I don't like to rely on sleeping pills as they make me feel groggy the next day, but a better routine and cutting out evening coffee and alcohol have definitely helped.*

As we have seen, poor sleep can have long-term effects for people who already have prediabetes or type 2 diabetes. Sleep is important for a number of brain functions, including how nerve cells (neurons) communicate. People who experience poor sleep or who do not get enough sleep find it harder to concentrate and respond quickly. They may be more likely to experience depression and may be at a higher risk of **Alzheimer's disease** or **dementia** later in life. If your sleep is irregular or poor, speak to your doctor for help in achieving better sleep to reduce your risk.

Smoking

Smoking is now proven to be an independent risk factor for insulin resistance and prediabetes, increasing the likelihood that type 2 diabetes will develop. Nicotine raises blood glucose levels, thickening the blood and increasing the risk of heart disease, stroke and circulatory problems, issues which are also associated with type 2 diabetes. This means that people who smoke are 30-40% more likely to develop type 2 than those who don't smoke. Elevated blood glucose levels are more difficult to control when nicotine is present and smoking damages the artery walls, making it easier for fatty deposits to build up, narrowing the vessels so a blood clot can develop. Quite simply, the more cigarettes you smoke, the greater your risk of type 2 diabetes.

Both smoking and high blood glucose levels in prediabetes and type 2 diabetes increase the risk of heart disease, so when these factors are combined the risk of damage to the circulatory system is increased dramatically. Both smoking and prediabetes lead to high glucose levels, because nicotine alters your body cells so they don't respond well to insulin, which increases blood glucose levels further, enabling fatty deposits to build up on your artery walls. As the arteries and blood vessels narrow the available space for blood to circulate is reduced, making it difficult for oxygenated blood to reach your hands and feet.

Poor blood supply can affect any part of the body. If the amount of oxygen that reaches the brain is reduced this can result in a stroke or heart attack if there is reduced blood flow to the coronary arteries of the heart. Smoking is a proven risk factor for insulin resistance which, if unrecognised and untreated, can eventually lead to premature death. Stopping smoking drastically reduces the risk of major complications related to high blood glucose levels.

> **FACT: There are 7000 chemicals in one cigarette.**

Remember that smoking increases blood glucose levels and insulin resistance. Nicotine in cigarettes, vapes and tobacco causes an inflammatory response in body cells, making it harder for these cells to use insulin correctly. Smoking more than 25 cigarettes a day can cause more body fat to accumulate around your middle and, even if you are not overweight, this central fat surrounds the abdominal organs, increasing the risk of insulin resistance and type 2 diabetes. Low-density (bad) **cholesterol** levels and triglyceride blood fats can also increase, while high-density lipoprotein or HDL (good) cholesterol levels go down. Elevated cholesterol and triglyceride levels are strongly linked to the development of type 2 diabetes.

Metabolic syndrome

Metabolic syndrome describes a group of associated conditions or risk factors that accompany type 2 diabetes, including obesity, coronary heart disease, high blood pressure, high blood fats (such as cholesterol) and high levels of chemicals that prevent the breakdown of blood clots in the arteries and heart. It is estimated that around one in four UK adults currently has metabolic syndrome.

Prediabetes is considered an underlying cause of metabolic syndrome, and having metabolic syndrome is a predictor of type 2 diabetes, heart and blood vessel disease, and stroke. This makes it sound as though metabolic syndrome and prediabetes are the same thing, but they are two separate and distinct health problems.

Metabolic syndrome covers a cluster of conditions that includes the symptoms of prediabetes. People with metabolic syndrome may have increased blood pressure, high blood glucose, excess fat around the waist, and high cholesterol and triglyceride levels, or only some of these factors. Although metabolic syndrome is typically associated with obesity, as many as one in five normal-weight adults can be at risk of prediabetes, too.

It is important to manage metabolic syndrome risk factors to prevent the development of prediabetes and coronary heart disease. The risk factors for metabolic syndrome are:

- Insulin resistance
- High blood pressure
- Being overweight or having obesity, especially visceral fat around the waist
- High triglycerides (a type of blood fat) combined with low HDL (good cholesterol).

Insulin resistance increases the risk of heart attack and stroke, high cholesterol levels also raise this risk, and having both insulin resistance and high cholesterol increases this risk even further. However, medicines can treat insulin resistance by lowering the amount of glucose released from your liver into your bloodstream and increasing the sensitivity of your body cells to insulin.

You may not currently have all the component risk factors that go towards a diagnosis of metabolic syndrome – perhaps you currently have obesity and high cholesterol levels, but not high blood pressure – and that means your increased risk of type 2 diabetes may be overlooked by health professionals. Having three or more of the risk factors I've listed suggests metabolic syndrome is present.

People who have metabolic syndrome are more likely to have prediabetes and type 2 diabetes. Factors such as obesity and a sedentary lifestyle play a major part in increasing the risk of developing prediabetes and then type 2 diabetes, so lifestyle changes are necessary to reverse this situation (for more on how to achieve lifestyle changes to improve your health, see Part II).

PETER SAYS: *I was diagnosed with metabolic syndrome last year. I had high levels of glucose in my blood, high cholesterol, high blood pressure and my weight was unhealthy, so I had quite a few of the risk factors. This was the first time I'd been to my doctor in a long time and it was for a routine health check. As I'm nearing 50, I realised it was time to take care of my health and I've now made several changes. I bought an exercise bike and use it every evening after my main meal. I've also halved the amount of alcohol I drink when socialising and aim to cut this further. I'm eating better foods, like brown rice and wholegrain bread instead of white, and cholesterol-lowering margarine instead of butter. After six months, I feel better, look better and my blood test results have drastically improved.*

High blood glucose levels

In association with long-term prediabetes, high blood glucose levels cause ongoing damage to the arteries, making them more likely to harden as the artery walls become stiff (**atherosclerosis**). Along with factors such as eating unhealthy foods, a lack of physical activity, regularly drinking alcohol and smoking, this can lead to high blood glucose and if high blood glucose is not controlled it can lead to sight problems, reduced kidney function, nerve disease, stroke and heart attack. Prediabetes is also linked to 'silent' or unrecognised heart attacks, where there is a blockage of blood flow to the heart and damage is done to the heart muscle.

High blood pressure

High blood pressure is a very common health problem. Blood pressure describes the amount of force exerted on blood vessel walls as blood is pumped around the body by the heart. High blood pressure means the heart has to work much harder to circulate blood around the body, putting increased strain on it. If there is also high blood glucose, this causes the blood to become sticky and thick, making it even more difficult to circulate and increasing the strain further.

> **❝ NAOMI SAYS:** *I had a doctor's appointment, because my head felt like it was going to explode with a constant pressure headache and my pulse was pounding away in my ears. The doctor diagnosed high blood pressure and gave me a prescription to lower it, but also did some other tests. My blood had too much glucose and on a second visit to get the results and assess my blood pressure again, I was told that I had prediabetes – which is associated with high blood pressure – and this was the cause of my problem. Although it didn't seem immediate enough, like prescribing some pills, my doctor advised me on lifestyle changes to help me lose some weight and be more active. I'm now trying to do more exercise and cut out salt wherever possible, because it's really bad for blood pressure, and salt is already added to so many foods you buy.* ❞

When blood pressure is recorded there are two numbers which indicate how well the heart is managing to pump blood. The **systolic blood pressure** (top number) records the pressure exerted on blood vessel walls at its peak as the heart beats. The **diastolic blood pressure** (bottom number) records the pressure on the vessel walls when the heart is at rest (blood pressure is at its lowest between beats). Both numbers provide useful information about blood pressure, but the systolic number is more important for diagnosing high blood pressure.

Blood pressure is measured in millilitres of mercury (mmHg):

- **Normal blood pressure**: Readings are anything between 90/60mmHg and 120/80mmHg.

- **Pre-high blood pressure**: Readings are between 120/80mmHg and 140/90mmHg.

- **High blood pressure**: Readings are consistently above 140/90mmHg. Also known as **hypertension**, it is diagnosed if you have three readings on three separate occasions when systolic pressure is 140 or above, diastolic pressure is 90 or above or both numbers are high each time.

Specific blood pressure targets for a person with diagnosed prediabetes or type 2 diabetes are usually below 140/90mmHg or below 150/90mmHg if you are 80 or older (for some people with kidney disease the target may be below 130/80mmHg).

MATT SAYS: *I was just mowing the front lawn one day when I began to feel dizzy and short of breath. Feeling really light-headed, I went to sit on the garden wall, not thinking anything of it. My neighbour came out and asked if I was OK. I said I was, but he told me I looked white as a sheet and offered to take me to hospital. It felt like a bit of an overreaction, but I agreed. An echocardiogram heart scan showed I had suffered a heart attack, but I was absolutely stunned, because there was no chest or arm pain and I'm only 42. The consultant said this is common – it's called a silent heart*

> *attack. It turns out that I also had high blood pressure and high glucose levels – another big surprise. I'm now trying to get fitter so it never happens again.*

A high sugar intake raises your blood glucose levels and thus your blood insulin levels, triggering your sympathetic nervous system to increase blood pressure and heart rate. That means reducing your sugar consumption is an effective way to reduce your blood pressure and therefore your risk of a range of health issues, including prediabetes and type 2 diabetes. Other lifestyle changes, such as cutting out salt and taking regular exercise, can also lower high blood pressure.

Where you live

While moving to another country to reduce your risk of developing type 2 diabetes isn't really realistic, the number of people with the condition is steadily rising in countries such as the UK and US. This is due to the increasing availability and consumption of high-fat, high-carbohydrate, high-calorie foods, and people living in Westernised countries also tend to be less physically active. Type 2 diabetes and its forerunner, prediabetes, are also becoming a serious issue in developing countries, where it is predicted that 70% of people aged 45 to 74 years will develop type 2 diabetes.

Although environment represents a moderate contribution to type 2 diabetes risk, where you live – climate, pollution levels and your access to healthy food options and green spaces – can affect your risk of developing the condition, and built-up, busy areas with a high degree of noise and air pollution are associated with a greater risk. The exact reason remains unclear, but this is probably due to the increased stress that these factors place on the body, and changes in these environmental factors may explain an increase in prediabetes and type 2 diabetes risk. In 2015, in the first research to quantify the contribution of air pollution to disease, tiny particles from car exhausts, wood burning stoves and industry were found to cause 14,900 new cases of type 2 diabetes per year. As air pollution continues to increase in towns and cities, cases of type 2 diabetes triggered by this risk are also set to rise.

✶ Key messages ✶

- Risk reduction is important because diabetes brings with it a number of serious secondary health conditions.

- Factors such as obesity and a sedentary lifestyle play a major part in increasing the risk of developing prediabetes and then type 2 diabetes.

- If you are overweight and have one or more of the risk factors described in this chapter, you should be tested for prediabetes.

- Being at risk does not necessarily mean you will definitely develop prediabetes or type 2 diabetes. However, taking steps to reduce certain risk factors will also benefit your overall health, such as your heart and circulatory system, so even a small change will make a big difference.

- People who smoke are 30-40% more likely to develop prediabetes and type 2 diabetes than those who don't smoke.

- Research shows that for those at high risk of developing prediabetes and type 2 diabetes, losing weight can reduce this risk by as much as 58% and regular exercise reduces the risk by 64%.

Chapter 4

Risk factors you can't control

This chapter takes a closer look at risk factors that cannot be controlled, but where awareness will allow you to manage your risk of prediabetes and type 2 diabetes.

Currently, one in nine adults has prediabetes. In fact, you may already have insulin resistance – where your body cells don't respond correctly to insulin and so can't use glucose effectively for fuel – but don't know it. Understanding the risk factors that increase your chances of developing prediabetes or type 2 diabetes is important, because it will probably make you more aware of changes in your health, which, in turn, will make early diagnosis more likely.

Fixed risk factors

Although these cannot be changed, there are six key risk factors that can increase your chances of developing prediabetes and type 2 diabetes. These are:

1. **Your age**: Being over 40 if you're white or over 35 if you're in a high-risk category.

2. **Your gender**: Being male – type 2 is slightly more common in men than women.

3. **Your ethnicity**: Being Afro-Caribbean, Black African or South Asian and also over 25.

4. **Your genetic inheritance**: Having a parent, sibling or child with type 2 diabetes.

5. **Your medical history**: Having certain conditions, including high blood pressure (now or in the past), heart disease or a stroke, **polycystic ovary syndrome** (PCOS), **non-alcoholic fatty liver disease** (NAFLD) or excess fat stored around your waistline.

6. **Gestational diabetes**: You have had the type of diabetes that develops during pregnancy.

There are also other factors that may contribute to insulin resistance, including:

- Medicines such as **glucocorticoids, antipsychotics** and some HIV treatments.
- Hormonal conditions such as **Cushing's syndrome**.
- Sleep disruption due to conditions such as **sleep apnoea**.

> **JOHN SAYS:** *My doctor tested my blood for prediabetes, because I'm overweight, 56 years old, and my brother and father already have type 2 diabetes. I wasn't feeling unwell or anything, but was surprised to find that my blood glucose levels were higher than they should be. This gave me the push to change what I could, like my weight. I knew this didn't mean I would definitely get diabetes one day, but it would be daft to put my head in the sand with a ticking time bomb. I've now taken action and started to exercise, and cut out processed sugary and fatty foods.*

The more risk factors that apply, the more likely it is that you will eventually develop prediabetes and type 2 diabetes. Having prediabetes not only means that you are more likely to develop type 2 diabetes at some stage, it also puts you at increased risk of heart disease and stroke. While this is a serious prospect, rest assured that although you will have factors like age that cannot be controlled, you can take steps to lower your overall risk by getting regular health checks, including blood glucose and blood pressure monitoring, working towards a healthy weight, getting regular exercise and taking prescribed medications to help reduce blood glucose and blood pressure levels.

> **FACT: Actor and filmmaker Tom Hanks says his type 2 diabetes is due to a mixture of genetics and a lifestyle of unhealthy eating. He tries to do an hour of exercise each day to manage the condition. When Tom was diagnosed in 2013, aged 57, his doctor told him, 'You know those high blood sugar numbers you've been dealing with since you were 36? Well, you've graduated. You've got type 2 diabetes, young man.'**

Am I at high risk?

As we saw in chapter 3, there are a number of reasons why type 2 diabetes risk is higher in some people than others. However, certain factors cannot be changed, so let's now have a look at these in more detail.

Age

After the age of 35, the risk of developing prediabetes and subsequently type 2 diabetes increases. If you're in a high-risk category, then you should ask your doctor for a blood test. If you're white, the age of 40 is often given for the general population, but the age is different for different ethnic groups so look at the section on ethnicity (*see* pp. 44–5). For young and middle-aged adults, it is important to know if you have prediabetes, because it's the precursor for type 2, but even if you can't change how old you are, it's definitely still worth making lifestyle changes to prevent or delay the development of full-blown type 2 diabetes.

Those who develop prediabetes and type 2 diabetes before the age of 40 tend to have the following factors in common:

- They have a greater degree of damage to the insulin-producing cells in their pancreas.
- They develop more complications due to high glucose because they have had prediabetes for a longer period before their type 2 diabetes is finally diagnosed.
- They tend to have a shorter lifespan than people of the same age without prediabetes or type 2 diabetes.

JEAN SAYS: *Aged 32, I began to feel tired and lethargic, with some blurry vision and headaches. I put it down to stress and computer screen time at work and home, and tried to sleep more. This didn't make things any better so I eventually visited my doctor, worrying that it was cancer, as these were the same symptoms a friend had with an operable brain tumour. My doctor arranged for some blood tests that showed I had high glucose levels on two different occasions. Although it's in my family, I was shocked to be diagnosed with prediabetes at such a young age. I thought it only happened to middle-aged and older people. Now, I'm determined to tackle this, so I don't get type 2 diabetes later on.*

Gender

Prediabetes and type 2 diabetes are more common in men, who are usually diagnosed at a younger age with a lower amount of body fat than women. Men tend to store more fat around the abdomen, which increases the risk of type 2 diabetes. It may be the case that men report any signs of prediabetes, like wounds that are slow to heal, less often or much later than women. Females with prediabetes or type 2 diabetes tend to develop more chronic complications from high blood glucose levels, such as eye and kidney problems, than men.

Men have an increased risk of developing type 2 diabetes when compared with women, and men aged 35 to 54 years are twice as likely to develop type 2 than women of that age. Most indicators of high blood glucose levels, such as thirst, increased urination and feeling tired, are the same in both genders. However, men particularly can experience a general reduction in muscle mass and erectile dysfunction when they have high glucose long term (for more on the complications that can occur over time, see chapter 5).

FACT: Over the past 12 years, rates of type 2 diabetes have risen four times faster in men aged 35 to 54 compared to women of the same age.

Men tend to already have cardiovascular disease as a risk factor for developing prediabetes and type 2 diabetes. Despite this specific gender-related risk for men, this does not mean that women should be any less watchful for any prediabetes indications. Type 2 tends to develop later in women, but heart disease as a consequence of long-term unrecognised and untreated high glucose levels is 50% more likely in women than men.

Ethnicity

Ethnicity increases the chance of developing prediabetes and type 2 diabetes because of family history (genetics) and social and environmental factors. From the age of 25, you are at increased risk of developing high glucose levels, followed by prediabetes and type 2, if you are from an Afro-Caribbean, Black African or South Asian (Indian, Pakistani, Bangladeshi) background.

Insulin resistance, where body cells don't respond correctly to insulin and cannot use glucose effectively for fuel, is more common in younger people from a South Asian background. As a result, Asian Indians are two to three times more likely to develop type 2 diabetes than other ethnic groups. It is thought this could be due to the way body fat is stored, particularly around the waistline. Fat deposits around the internal organs (visceral fat), such as the liver and pancreas, increase insulin resistance, elevate blood glucose levels and raise the risk of developing type 2 diabetes.

> **FACT: Be aware of your increased risk. As we have already seen, as long as you are aware, your increased type 2 diabetes risk can be managed and in many cases delayed.**

Prediabetes and type 2 diabetes are more common in some ethnic groups than others. American Indians develop type 2 at nearly twice the rate Caucasians do. Latinos, Asians and African Americans are also at higher risk.

❝ **ZAHOOR SAYS:** *I've been told I have a higher chance of developing type 2 diabetes because of my Bangladeshi ethnicity. This shocked me and I thought about it for a long time before deciding that, although I can't change this, I can change my lifestyle in a few ways. I want to lower my chance of getting diabetes in any way I can because several of my relatives have it and it causes other serious health problems. I also have an older brother who has to take tablets to lower his sugar levels, although he hasn't got diabetes yet. So far, I've stopped smoking and cut out sugary foods and takeaways. That's just the start. I also plan to start exercising to get my weight down and get fitter. It's more difficult to try and make several changes at the same time, so I have a better chance of success by doing it in stages. Diabetes prevention is now my incentive and motivation.* ❞

Genetics

Prediabetes can develop due to a genetic predisposition that is impacted by lifestyle factors. Even people who exercise, eat well and maintain a normal weight can develop prediabetes if they have a genetic risk that increases the chance of developing the condition. Type 2 diabetes mostly results from genetic, environmental and other factors combined, but if you have a parent, sibling or child with type 2, it greatly increases your chances of developing the condition, too. The level of risk is as follows:

- 15% if either your mother or father has prediabetes or type 2 diabetes.
- 75% if both your mother and father have prediabetes or type 2 diabetes.
- 10% if your non-identical twin has prediabetes or type 2 diabetes.
- 90% if your identical twin has prediabetes or type 2 diabetes.

The risk of developing type 2 is higher if your mother rather than your father has prediabetes or type 2 diabetes. Prediabetes and type 2 diabetes are therefore only partly inherited, with first-degree relatives being more likely to develop these conditions than those who do not have type 2 in their family. There are also other kinds of diabetes that are directly inherited from your parents, such as **maturity onset diabetes** (MODY) in young people and diabetes that is due to a DNA mutation.

KAVITA SAYS: *My mum had gestational diabetes when she was pregnant with me, then she developed type 2 diabetes seven years later. My dad also developed type 2, because it was common in his family. My sister has had type 1 diabetes since the age of 10 and I feel as though I've inherited a ticking time bomb for diabetes. I'm hyper-aware of it and base my lifestyle around it – I keep my weight at a sensible level* *and eat healthy foods with the knowledge that diabetes is just around the corner and will arrive more quickly if I don't watch out. I also exercise regularly and I don't smoke. I know I have a high genetic risk of developing type 2 someday, so I have yearly blood glucose tests and I'm doing all I can to delay the onset of prediabetes.*

As we have seen, type 2 diabetes is in part inherited. Despite this, neither prediabetes or full-blown type 2 is completely due to genetic factors. If you are at increased risk, environmental factors can trigger and accelerate the onset of high blood glucose levels due to insulin resistance. Several genes in the DNA are known as susceptibility genes. A person with these genes is at higher risk of developing prediabetes and type 2 diabetes, because they are more susceptible than someone without these genetic factors. People without diabetes also have a greater immunity to prediabetes and type 2 due to other genes.

MARIA SAYS: *I was on holiday in Greece with my sister Jean. We did a lot of walking, which we both enjoy, but I felt tired, headachy and my brain was a bit fuzzy. I'm 52 and assumed the symptoms were the menopause, so I carried on, but had a nap in the afternoons when it was really hot.*

When we got home I booked an appointment with the practice nurse – my doctor is male and I didn't particularly want to discuss the menopause with him – but when I described my symptoms to her, she said I would need to provide a urine sample and have a blood test. I couldn't understand why, but didn't ask, thinking it must be to test hormone levels. The tests showed a high amount of glucose in my blood and I was told to come back to the surgery for another quick blood test a few days later.

The nurse said she couldn't tell me anything until they had the results of the second blood test and then I might have to see the doctor. This made me very anxious and I'd worked myself up into quite a state when I went for the second test. When I was finally called in to see the doctor he told me quite simply, "You have type 2 diabetes."

I couldn't really process this information and the doctor gave me a few moments before explaining that my symptoms were from high sugars, not the menopause, and I had probably developed type 2 diabetes because of a genetic risk and lifestyle factors. Jean was waiting for me outside in the car. I got in and told her the diagnosis. She nodded and said, "I thought it would be diabetes, just like me."

Jean takes it all in her stride, managing the condition really well and living a full and happy life. With her guidance and support, I've adapted quickly to doing things slightly differently. I control my carbohydrate portions and make sure I take exercise to keep my blood glucose levels in check, and I know that if I don't, I could experience low mood. I also take a diabetes medicine by mouth. It's an alternative to metformin, which wasn't suitable for me.

What I'd say to anyone with symptoms is get them checked at the earliest opportunity and don't make excuses that they are related to age or the menopause. I'd also say don't let having diabetes stop you from leading the life you want to live.

Medical history

There are a number of medical conditions associated with prediabetes and type 2 diabetes:

- **High blood pressure**: This is significant whether you currently have it or have ever had it.

- **Heart disease or a stroke**: These conditions share common risk factors with type 2 diabetes, such as high blood pressure and high cholesterol.

- *Polycystic ovary syndrome* **(PCOS)**: With this condition your ovaries contain a large number of harmless follicles where eggs develop but cannot be released, so ovulation does not take place.

- **Non-alcoholic fatty liver disease (NAFLD)**: This affects the amount of fat in the liver, which can interfere with how your body uses glucose.

- **Excess fat stored around your waistline**: This accumulates around the liver and pancreas, causing insulin resistance, because the insulin in your body can't work properly.

- **Thyroid dysfunction**: This can affect your metabolism and your insulin function, and, in particular, low levels of thyroid hormone (*hypothyroidism*) can impair the production and uptake of insulin, leading to higher blood glucose levels.

- **Growth hormone**: At elevated levels this can lead to insulin resistance as growth hormone hinders the action of insulin and promotes glucose production in the liver. Excess **cortisol** (the stress hormone) can also lead to insulin resistance and high blood glucose levels.

- **Schizophrenia**: The association relates to behaviour patterns, such as too little exercise, stress, poor sleep, smoking and an unhealthy diet, and therefore high cholesterol, leading to elevated blood glucose levels. Antipsychotic schizophrenia medicines, such as clozapine and olanzapine, can also increase the risk of type 2 diabetes.

- **Bipolar disorder**: As with schizophrenia, lifestyle is a contributing factor.
- **Depression**: There is evidence that depression is more common in people with prediabetes and in those with undiagnosed prediabetes.

Diabetes and depression

There is a close association between depression and diabetes, and some of the symptoms, such as tiredness, are similar. When a person has depression, their blood glucose levels tend to be higher than normal, so type 2 diabetes can develop following a period of depression. However, if someone has high blood glucose levels, they are also more likely to become depressed, partly because of inflammation and hormone imbalance, but also because self-managing diabetes can be difficult and stressful in itself, leading to depression (see chapter 8 for more on emotional health).

Depression is often overlooked as a result of diabetes, but if you have diabetes and think you may be depressed, see your doctor, because treatment may help you to adopt the necessary lifestyle changes that will help to reverse your prediabetes or type 2 diabetes and, in turn, your depressive symptoms.

> **ROBYN SAYS:** *I can't even say that one thing in particular was the problem, just that everything seemed to be too much effort and I couldn't be bothered. My family encouraged me to go to my doctor, who listened and prescribed antidepressants. What he didn't do, though, was diagnose prediabetes. After a few months on the tablets, I agreed to walk to the supermarket with a friend. There was a Diabetes UK tent in the car park and they were testing people's blood. They invited me to have the test and I decided I would do it. Just as well – the result suggested I had prediabetes. After finding on the internet that depression is associated*

with high blood sugar, this was the motivation I needed to help myself to a healthier lifestyle. I saw my doctor again the following week.

Hormonal conditions

Some hormonal conditions cause the body to produce increased amounts of certain hormones, which can lead to type 2 diabetes. Cushing's syndrome, for example, occurs when the body produces too much stress hormone (cortisol), which in turn increases blood glucose and blood pressure. Similarly, **acromegaly**, when the body produces too much growth hormone, can also cause insulin resistance, leading to increases in blood glucose levels.

The hormonal changes associated with menopause, which normally occurs between the ages of 45 and 55, can also cause some women's blood pressure to increase and some women to gain weight. Menopause is prompted by reduced production of the hormone **oestrogen**, and the change in oestrogen production and increase in fat stored around the middle of the body leads to insulin resistance, resulting in higher blood glucose levels, because insulin cannot work properly.

With the associated lower levels of oestrogen production, and increasing risk factors affecting blood pressure and body weight, avoiding prediabetes during and after menopause can be challenging. If you are a smoker, giving up will help your body use insulin more effectively, as will eating a healthy diet and keeping active (*see Part II for ways to implement healthy and achievable lifestyle changes*).

GILL SAYS: *I thought I was feeling not quite right because I'd started the menopause six months earlier, so I didn't report it to my doctor. I saw a nurse for something else and just mentioned that I felt tired and had regular headaches. She measured my blood pressure, which was up, and did a finger-prick blood test that showed my cholesterol and glucose levels were also high. I came away from that* *appointment in disbelief that suddenly my health was failing and all because of the menopause. Suddenly, I had prediabetes and was at increased risk of heart disease and stroke. I then saw my (male) doctor, who prescribed statins and lifestyle change, although I was expecting hormone replacement treatment. When I asked, he said all women go through the menopause and although my symptoms were most likely due to reduced oestrogen levels, he would not prescribe hormone replacement as I couldn't remain on it for the rest of my life.*

Gestational diabetes

Gestational diabetes is a type of diabetes that can develop during pregnancy in women who don't already have any other form of diabetes. The condition occurs because a hormone made by the placenta prevents the body from using insulin effectively, causing glucose to build up in the blood instead of being absorbed by the cells. Blood glucose levels vary far more than normal during pregnancy due to hormonal variations and gestational diabetes makes this worse.

LORNA SAYS: *I had a lot of problems with gestational diabetes when I had my second child. I was hospitalised several times with really high glucose levels and the metabolic effects of this (ketoacidosis). I ate a special low-carbohydrate diet, took exercise regularly, tested my blood glucose several times a day and also had to take insulin injections. Despite this, the high glucose meant my baby weighed 12 pounds and had to be born by Caesarean section. Thankfully the baby was fine and survived without any ill effects, but six years later I developed type 2 diabetes as a consequence of having an altered metabolism during pregnancy.*

Unlike type 1 diabetes, gestational diabetes is not caused by a lack of insulin, but by other hormones produced during pregnancy that create insulin resistance, making insulin less effective. Some of the reasons why gestational diabetes occurs may include being overweight or having obesity, having previously given birth to a baby weighing more than nine pounds and a family history of type 2 diabetes.

Women usually have normal blood glucose levels in the first trimester of pregnancy and gestational diabetes may only be discovered in the second or third trimester during a routine blood test. There is no definitive blood glucose level to confirm gestational diabetes, but it is diagnosed if regular tests show a consistently elevated blood glucose level (this usually disappears after the baby is born). However, more than half of mothers who have had gestational diabetes will go on to develop type 2 diabetes within 15 years.

> **FACT: Two London hospitals are using AI to spot type 2 diabetes risk up to 10 years before it is usually diagnosed. Imperial College and Chelsea and Westminster Hospital NHS Foundation Trusts are training AI systems, known as Aire-AI, to check electrocardiogram (ECG) heart traces and early results suggest that AI could also detect who is at risk of type 2 diabetes 70% of the time.**

Even though there are factors you cannot control, the good news is that there are ways to delay a diagnosis of prediabetes or type 2 diabetes for as long as possible, and perhaps prevent it altogether. You'll find all the information, advice and support you need to help you change what is possible and manage what can't be changed in Part II.

✷ Key messages ✷

- People who are white and over the age of 40 are at increased risk of developing prediabetes and type 2 diabetes. If you are in a high-risk category, you should have a blood test when you're 35.

- From the age of 25, you are at increased risk of developing prediabetes and type 2 diabetes if you are from an Afro-Caribbean, Black African or South Asian background.

- Men aged 35 to 54 years are twice as likely to develop prediabetes and type 2 diabetes than women of that age.

- Some older people may not be able to produce adequate amounts of insulin when they eat, due to ageing of the insulin-producing cells in the pancreas, meaning that lifestyle factors are not always the reason for prediabetes and type 2 diabetes.

- Although it is possible to develop type 2 diabetes at any age, the risk of prediabetes increases after the age of 35.

- Although you may not currently have any risk factors other than age, it is important to be tested for prediabetes once you reach 40 years of age.

Chapter 5

Chronic complications

This chapter focuses on the secondary health problems – which are known as complications – caused by unrecognised or untreated high blood glucose levels

Although we need glucose for fuel so the body can function normally, too much glucose has a negative effect on cells and is actually toxic above certain levels. If you have prediabetes or type 2 diabetes and it is undiagnosed, and therefore remains untreated, the high levels of glucose in your blood alter the way your body can use glucose. Eventually this damages the structure of the cells in your body, affecting how they work. This means that over time high blood glucose levels – when there is too little insulin, or when the body can't use insulin properly (for more on how this works, see chapter 1) – are very damaging, particularly if you don't realise you have them.

What to look out for

The symptoms of prediabetes and type 2 diabetes, like an unquenchable thirst and frequent urination (for more on symptoms, see chapter 2), are short-term indicators that you have high blood glucose levels, while complications are the long-term consequences of unrecognised or untreated high blood glucose levels.

Many people with newly diagnosed type 2 diabetes already have complications like heart disease and/or nerve damage, so if you spot any changes in your health, tell your doctor as soon as possible. I'm pleased to say, though, that if you report these as soon as you notice them, the deterioration can be significantly reduced. Here, I'm going to look at eight serious complications of undiagnosed or long-term high blood glucose levels. They are:

1. **Sight problems**: You may develop blurred vision, floaters, blind spots or notice a halo around bright lights.

2. **Reduced kidney function**: You may produce more or less urine than normal and, if it's less, the urine will be darker in colour. You may feel constantly tired, itchy, irritable, have a constant headache or often feel sick.

3. **Impaired nerve function**: You may feel burning, numbness or tingling in your feet, legs and hands. When you walk it might seem like you're walking on pebbles, or you may not realise that you've cut yourself or have a blister. You may also notice that you can no longer feel pain, heat or cold.

4. **Heart disease**: This may present as shortness of breath or a tight chest, and you may feel pain and discomfort. You may feel tired, have dizzy spells or feel as though your heartbeat is very weak or irregular.

5. **Circulatory problems**: Symptoms of reduced circulation are closely linked to symptoms of nerve damage (see p. 62), and you may experience cold hands and/or feet, and slow wound healing.

6. **Foot problems**: Pain when you put pressure on your feet and hard skin build-up are a common early sign of complications caused

by high blood glucose levels. You may have noticed that you can't detect hot, cold or sharp sensations with your feet, feel numbness and cold, and prickling at night. Any cuts/scratches/sores or blisters are slow to heal.

7. **Gum disease**: You may notice bleeding when you brush your teeth and your gums may be tender, sore or swollen. You may also have bad breath or loose teeth.

8. **Sexual problems**: These are common, due to nerve damage and reduced blood supply. Men may experience erectile dysfunction, while women may have vaginal dryness and pain on intercourse. Low libido (sex drive) can affect both men and women.

Close-up on long-term issues

Because high blood glucose and prediabetes can take 10 years or more to finally be diagnosed, by the time they receive their diagnosis, 72% of people have already developed significant problems. That's why it's so important to be aware of what those secondary health conditions are. More information on the complications that can arise from diabetes follows, including what you can do if you spot any additional symptoms.

Sight problems

If you experience any of the following changes in your vision, then it is important to visit your doctor or an optician, who can refer you to an ophthalmologist (eye doctor) if necessary. Signs that high blood glucose levels are affecting your sight can include:

- Blurry vision
- Eye floaters
- Blind spots
- A halo around bright lights.

Noticing that your sight has become blurry may be the first indication of persistently elevated glucose levels, but fortunately even when it is advanced, damage to the eyes caused by high glucose levels doesn't always cause major sight loss. It is the case, though, that a high-carbohydrate diet in association with insufficient insulin production is a bad combination over time, causing damage to the tiny blood vessels at the back of the eye and potential sight problems.

There are several eye conditions associated with prolonged high blood glucose levels:

- Retinopathy: An association between high glucose levels and damage to the retina has long been recognised in people with undiagnosed and diagnosed prediabetes and type 2 diabetes. **Retinopathy** describes changes to the blood vessels supplying the retina at the back of each eye. Elevated blood glucose can cause these vessels to leak and new blood vessels to form on the retinal surface, affecting vision. Retinopathy can be treated, but the best way to preserve your sight is to prevent retinopathy from happening in the first place by reducing and maintaining healthy blood glucose levels.

- Macular oedema: A **macular oedema** describes swelling of the macula – the area at the centre of the retina that provides sharp, straight vision – causing blurred or distorted vision. A further eye condition that is common in people with prolonged **hyperglycaemia** (high glucose levels) is **macular degeneration**. This leads to a loss of central vision and is usually associated with older age, although a diet rich in white carbohydrates (white bread, white rice, white pasta) and resulting high glucose levels over time may trigger onset at an earlier age.

- Cataracts: They form due to protein deposits which cause a clouding of the lens – the clear part of the eye that helps to focus light – affecting central vision. After the age of 40, proteins in the lens of the eye naturally start to break down. Most **cataracts** happen because of these natural changes over time. However, cataracts appear at an earlier age and progress faster in people who have had prolonged hyperglycaemia.

- Glaucoma: Elevated blood glucose levels increase swelling, which raises eye pressure, narrows blood vessels and eventually becomes the eye condition glaucoma. One form of **glaucoma – neovascular**

glaucoma – is the result of high glucose levels damaging the surface of the retina at the back of the eye. This condition causes bleeding, raising eye pressure to encourage new and abnormal blood vessels to grow on the iris (the coloured part of the eye), which increases eye pressure further.

If you experience blurred vision, the appearance of rings around lights or dark spots, sensitivity to sunlight and other bright lights, trouble seeing at night or difficulty reading, you should visit an ophthalmologist. You can do a lot to help your eye health by having yearly eye checks, eating a healthy diet, taking regular exercise and giving up smoking to normalise blood glucose levels and prevent 90% of eye disease. However, if you do experience any sight changes, the sooner you visit an eye specialist, the better.

JAN SAYS: *I went to my optician for new glasses and was shocked to be told that, at the age of 38, I had the beginnings of a cataract forming in one eye and increased eye pressure. I then found out that this could have been triggered by my poor diet, because I do have a sweet tooth and didn't eat a particularly healthy diet. My doctor did a couple of blood tests and told me I had borderline type 2 diabetes, advising me on diet and exercise changes I should make. So, I've now given up the sweet stuff and joined an exercise class to prevent my eyesight from getting any worse.*

Reduced kidney function

The following are signs that elevated glucose levels could have affected your kidneys, and if you spot any of the following changes, you should report them to your doctor as soon as possible to get a proper diagnosis:

- Different urination patterns – needing to go more or less often
- Noticing your urine is consistently darker in colour or foamy

- Swollen ankles
- Tightness in your chest
- Always feeling tired
- Itchiness
- Being irritable
- Having a constant headache
- Often feeling sick.

When your blood glucose levels are higher than normal, your kidneys have to work much harder to filter glucose from your blood, leading to a greater volume of urine and a need to urinate more frequently. The higher the concentration of glucose in the blood, the more that is passed in the urine as the body attempts to get rid of this excess. Each kidney is made up of millions of tiny filtration units called nephrons. High blood glucose levels can damage these nephrons, as well as the blood vessels in your kidneys, so they don't work as well as they should.

Excess glucose in the bloodstream can cause the kidneys to filter too much blood. Over time, this extra work affects the function of the nephrons, often resulting in the loss of their vital filtering ability. If this occurs continuously over months or even longer, the larger glucose molecules that have passed through the nephrons into your urine cause lasting damage to the structure of your kidneys, although this does not cause any pain. Unfortunately, reduced kidney function may not be detected in tests until the deterioration is significantly advanced.

However, although there are often no early warning signs of kidney disease (**nephropathy**), the later stages can be controlled with medicines that reduce blood glucose levels and also blood pressure, as high blood pressure can accelerate the damage. These medicines are effective at significantly reducing the risk of kidney failure.

SHELLEY SAYS: *I had no idea there was anything wrong as I had no pain to suggest a kidney problem. However, over a period of months I noticed that my legs and feet felt* *uncomfortably swollen and tight. I was also having muscle cramps in my right arm and left calf, plus dry, itchy skin on my legs. As time went on, I began to get short of breath without physically exerting myself, although I also have asthma, so I put it down to that. I didn't have much of an appetite and noticed I was visiting the loo less frequently. I also started to have problems with my eyesight, with blurred vision and some blind spots. Again, I put it down to other things, because I've always worn glasses and assumed I needed a new prescription. When I finally reported all this to my doctor, he suspected impaired kidney function and he investigated this further. I now take medicines to stabilise the damage caused by high glucose levels.*

Impaired nerve function

The circulatory and/or nerve problems listed below may indicate you have prediabetes or type 2 diabetes, and if you notice any of the following nerve changes, tell your doctor:

- Prickling, pain or numbness in your hands, feet or legs
- Weakness in your arms or legs
- Nerve pain
- Reduced or lost pain or sensation, or decreased ability to feel heat or cold, in your feet
- You may feel as though you are walking on pebbles
- Dizziness or light-headedness
- Ongoing stomach problems like nausea, vomiting or diarrhoea
- Repeated bladder infections or trouble emptying your bladder
- Problems having or sustaining an erection.

Sometimes, nerve damage – known as **neuropathy** – can be the first sign of long-term elevated glucose levels. This condition is also more likely to occur in those over 40 years of age and in people who smoke. Neuropathy can affect different nerves in the body, especially those in the feet and hands, organs and muscles, and there are different types of neuropathies:

- **Peripheral neuropathy**: This affects the hands, arms, feet and legs, causing pain, numbness, tingling and weakness.
- **Sensory neuropathy**: This results in a loss of sensation in different areas of the body.
- **Autonomic neuropathy**: This affects the function of internal organs, such as the bladder, digestive system and heart.
- **Motor neuropathy**: This is a progressive muscle disorder characterised by weakness in different muscles.

A particular type of nerve damage due to ongoing high blood glucose levels can affect your stomach and bowels, causing continuing diarrhoea or constipation; bladder, causing urinary incontinence; genitals, causing vaginal dryness, poor libido and erectile dysfunction; and heart, causing disruption to your heart rhythm. Neuropathy can affect any part of the nervous system throughout the body, but as with all complications due to high blood glucose levels, this can be reversed or significantly improved with lifestyle changes (see Part II).

HANNAH SAYS: *I had stomach trouble for over a year and finally went to my doctor because I had lost weight and the diarrhoea wasn't going away. I thought it was an ongoing stomach bug or food poisoning, and scrubbed out my fridge with bleach in case I was reinfecting myself. When I had blood tests, though, they showed that it wasn't an infection causing the issue. I had high blood glucose levels and because I didn't get the symptoms checked earlier, the nerve damage in my gut is permanent. I now take meds for type 2 diabetes.*

Peripheral neuropathy in the hands and feet can be improved by reducing blood glucose levels. Your doctor may prescribe an anticonvulsant medicine, which is often used for nerve pain, or creams or patches to be applied to your skin. A portable TENS (transcutaneous electrical stimulation) machine, which is available from larger pharmacies, may also help. This device stimulates the nerves and reduces pain signals.

> **LIV SAYS:** *I've got prediabetes, and peripheral and autonomic neuropathy, and it rules my life. Peripheral neuropathy in my feet is worse at night and burns like a hot wire pushed under the skin. When I walk it feels like I'm walking across pebbles, and it's painful and uncomfortable. This has all been caused by high glucose levels going unchecked for years. The autonomic neuropathy has affected the nerves controlling my heart and digestion. I can't eat much without feeling terribly bloated and uncomfortable for hours afterwards, and it took a long time to be diagnosed because I was told I had irritable bowel syndrome for several years when it was really constant diarrhoea due to autonomic neuropathy. I have cardiac arrhythmia, where heartbeats are missed due to nerve damage. I'm now controlling my blood glucose and these problems have improved a lot, so I'd like to tell people to get checked early for other health problems and start feeling the health benefits of reducing glucose levels.*

Heart disease

As I've already said, you should report changes in your overall health to your doctor, but high blood glucose levels can often cause damage to the heart and circulatory system, so if you experience any of the following signs it is particularly important to speak to your doctor, as they may indicate issues with your heart health:

- Shortness of breath or a tight chest
- Chest pain and discomfort on exertion (known as **angina pectoris**)

- Dizzy spells
- Feeling tired
- As though your heartbeat is very weak or irregular
- Cold limbs
- Recurrent chest pain.

Unfortunately, heart disease and elevated blood glucose levels are inextricably linked. Over time, even slightly raised glucose levels can start to damage blood vessels. When your body can no longer use glucose properly for fuel, more glucose sticks to your red blood cells, altering their capacity to carry oxygen. This glucose build-up can block and damage the vessels carrying blood to and from the heart, reducing the available supply of oxygen and nutrients.

Other risk factors include high blood pressure and blood fats, changes in the way the blood clots and an increase in the level of insulin in the blood as your body tries to reverse the high levels of glucose. This is also associated with an increase in fatty deposits inside the arteries, encouraging blood clot formation.

Fatty deposits in the blood – cholesterol – can stick to the artery walls, especially those around the heart. This is known as atherosclerosis and it's the most common cause of a heart attack. Over time this fat hardens and is known as **plaque**. These arteries become narrow and restrict the amount of blood that flows through them. This can cause chest pain on exertion. In these narrowed blood vessels blood flow is slower, causing blood cells to group together and easily form a clot. If the clot breaks away it will travel through the arteries and veins until it cannot pass through and is stopped by another narrowed vessel, resulting in a partial or complete blockage that severely reduces or stops blood flow completely. The heart is then starved of oxygen, resulting in a heart attack.

High levels of glucose also thicken the blood – think of syrup being pumped around a radiator – putting further strain on the heart and arteries, in addition to the presence of blood fats, such as cholesterol, narrowing the walls of your arteries. If you have high blood pressure as well that is yet another strain on heart and blood vessels that are already affected by atherosclerosis.

There are 7.4 million people in the UK currently living with heart and circulatory problems, but lifestyle changes (see Part II) are a positive and effective way to reduce and prevent heart and artery disease.

BARRY SAYS: *I was actually at my daughter's wedding when I had pains in my left arm and tightness in my chest. I thought it was the stress of the event, so I sat at the reception for about an hour and said nothing, not wanting to upstage the bride. My brother told me I looked pale and sweaty, and insisted I went to hospital. After some tests, the senior emergency doctor asked why I hadn't told him I had type 2 diabetes. I was absolutely shocked. I'm 42 and had no idea I had diabetes. I can honestly say there were no symptoms, like drinking and urinating more, and there's no family history of type 2 diabetes. The consultant said the heart attack was due to the diabetes being present for a few years. The hospital gave me great advice and support for lifestyle changes: regular exercise, eating well and keeping my blood glucose under control.*

Circulatory problems

You may have noticed a cut, bruise or blister on your skin that is taking a long time to heal. High blood glucose levels thicken the blood and cause it to circulate more slowly. This makes it difficult for the body to deliver essential healing nutrients to wounds. The symptoms of reduced circulation, such as slow wound healing and cold hands and/or feet, are closely linked to the symptoms of nerve damage (see pp. 61–3), although circulatory problems affecting the large blood vessels in your legs may first become noticeable through cramps, changes in skin colour and reduced sensation.

A partial narrowing of the arteries supplying the brain may result in a 'mini stroke' (**transient ischaemic attack**). Common symptoms of a transient ischaemic attack include your face dropping on one side, not being able to lift your arms and speech problems. Several of these episodes can lead to a full stroke. Although high blood glucose levels are not their only cause, by taking action to reduce your blood pressure and levels of blood fats, as well as your blood glucose, you can lower your risk of mini-stroke and full stroke.

Unfortunately, having prolonged high glucose levels also increases the risk of developing vascular disease or disease that affects the blood vessels. **Peripheral vascular disease** is the reduced circulation of blood to a body part other than the brain or heart and it's caused by narrowed or blocked blood vessels. The main cause of this condition is atherosclerosis, which, as I have explained, is the build-up of fatty deposits that narrow a blood vessel, usually within an artery. This can affect multiple arteries and blood vessels, including those in the heart, neck and leg, and may occur due to long-term undiagnosed high glucose levels, as well as genetic factors and ageing.

> **ARJUN SAYS:** *My feet and hands feel numb and cold all the time, even when the heating is turned up. My doctor said this is due to poor circulation and he did some tests to find out why. The blood tests showed quite a high glucose result and because I also have high blood pressure and I'm overweight, I had more tests on my heart. This showed narrowing in the arteries – all very worrying and quite a shock to find out. I'm now losing weight with a local slimming group and I do exercise classes with my brother, who also wants to lose weight, so we give each other support. The aim is to get healthier and avoid a heart attack, which was our father's cause of death.*

Unfortunately, blood vessel damage in association with nerve damage can cause foot problems that, at their most serious, can lead to amputation. Circulatory problems will result in reduced blood supply in your feet and this poor blood supply means problems with cuts, bruises, blisters and sores not healing. The good news is that reducing blood glucose levels with a healthy diet and regular exercise can avoid these problems, or stop them from getting worse.

FACT: Mark Labbett – the Beast on UK TV quiz *The Chase* – only discovered he had diabetes after the skin on his legs failed to heal. A nurse noticed this and suggested he might have type 2 diabetes, which was confirmed by a blood test.

Foot problems

Foot problems are a common early sign of high blood glucose levels in either diagnosed or undiagnosed prediabetes and type 2 diabetes, and I make no apology for saying it again: report any changes in your feet to your doctor as soon as you notice them.

Typically, at first you may experience a loss of feeling or slight numbness or tingling in your toes. This can progress and eventually you may be less able to feel pain or pressure or detect temperature differences. You may experience prickling pain with hard skin build-up or even flashing pains that go from your feet up into your lower legs. Raised blood glucose levels damage nerves controlling the sensations in your feet and the motor nerves affecting balance, as well as impacting blood circulation, which leads to a reduced blood supply to the lower limbs. It is important to check your feet daily for any changes, as you may not feel them, especially if you have a hard area of skin that has formed from the pressure of a shoe (or rubbing of a sock), or a wound or blister on your foot that is slow to heal.

DAVE SAYS: *I realised that very gradually my feet had become progressively numb and cold, and I started wearing two pairs of socks. I considered myself relatively healthy, so thought nothing of it. Then, one day, I trod on something hard in bare feet after getting out of the shower and noticed that it didn't hurt. A few days later, I saw a cut on the bottom of one foot that had become infected and I hadn't realised there was a wound. I dressed the injury and assumed it would heal; it didn't. After five months and several courses of antibiotics, a blood test confirmed that I had prediabetes. My foot is now*

> *healing slowly with blood glucose-reducing medication, but my doctor said things would have been very different if I'd left the wound any longer and kept walking on it.* 🙸

As we can see from Dave's experience, damage to the nerves in the feet can result in a reduced ability to detect cuts and blisters on the feet, which may become infected and lead to a foot ulcer. Constant pressure from part of a shoe on a particular area of the foot may not be detected either. Over time an area of hard protective skin then develops. Continued pressure on the hardened skin causes it to soften, become mushy and eventually break down, leaving a deep hole or ulcer that can become infected. This can take a long time to heal or may not heal at all. An untreated foot ulcer like this can, at its most serious, lead to amputation. Again, as with all long-term complications caused by high blood glucose over a period of time, the key is to change your lifestyle and reduce blood glucose to a healthy level.

Gum disease

Gum disease is common when you have high blood glucose levels. If your blood has high levels of glucose, all your body fluids will be high in glucose, too, which means that your saliva attracts more bacteria, and your teeth and gums are targeted by it. Report any of the following to your dentist or doctor as soon as possible:

- Gums that are sore and bleed easily after brushing and flossing
- Gums that are swollen, red and tender
- Gaps between the gum and the tooth
- Prolonged bad breath
- Loose teeth.

Gum disease is an infection of the tissues surrounding and supporting the teeth. It is more likely when glucose levels are persistently raised and it is usually associated with the build-up of plaque (a sticky film). It won't improve if blood glucose levels remain elevated as bacteria in the plaque feed off the glucose, producing more plaque. Some of these bacteria can cause tooth decay, cavities and gum disease, and if the tooth isn't treated, it can also lead to tooth loss. In addition, elevated blood glucose levels mean there is less saliva in the mouth to protect against bacteria.

When bacteria in plaque are plentiful in the mouth they can enter the bloodstream. Oral bacteria can then migrate through the blood, from the mouth to the arterial plaques, worsening artery disease (atherosclerosis) and over time causing steady damage to the heart, blood vessels and brain. Visit your dentist regularly and take good care of your teeth each day by brushing, flossing and rinsing with an antiseptic mouthwash to reduce oral bacteria. However, the dietary and lifestyle changes that will protect your teeth will also help keep your blood glucose under control (see Part II).

Sexual problems

Sexual problems are common in people with prediabetes and type 2 diabetes. Men may experience erectile dysfunction – many men only discover they have type 2 diabetes because they have erectile dysfunction and go to the doctor. Women may have vaginal dryness, irritation and pain on intercourse. Low libido can affect both men and women.

High glucose levels and elevated cholesterol over time can affect the sexual health and function of both men and women. Prolonged high glucose affects the function of nerves and blood vessels that supply the sexual organs. Reduced blood flow can result in a loss of feeling in these areas and reduced sexual desire. High blood glucose levels also affect the production of the hormone testosterone, which is often a reason for sexual dysfunction in both men and women.

DAN SAYS: *I began noticing erectile problems and I was always tired. I put this down to work pressures and tried not to dwell on it too much. After several months my wife suggested I see my doctor. He said the problem was common and often due to stress or alcohol consumption, but he did some blood tests just to be sure there was no underlying cause. It turns out I have elevated blood glucose levels and erectile dysfunction is a complication of that. I was completely shocked and have* *made some lifestyle changes to tackle the high glucose levels. I'm taking medication now which has helped the erectile dysfunction, but I hope to stop this once my weight and glucose levels are under control. I believe in tackling the root cause of any health problem rather than just taking pills to treat it, if possible.*

Other warning signs

Skin problems like yeast infections are another warning that blood glucose is too high, as yeast loves to feed on glucose (yeast derives energy by fermenting sugars and carbohydrates). Symptoms to look out for are itching in moist areas, such as armpits, under the breasts, and between fingers and toes. For women, a yeast infection can cause vaginal discharge, itching and pain. For uncircumcised men, a yeast infection may cause itching around the foreskin. If you have frequent yeast infections, your doctor will prescribe medicine to treat this and order a blood test to check your glucose levels.

Other skin-related symptoms of high blood glucose include hair loss on the toes, feet and lower legs, and brown patches of raised skin on the sides and back of your neck, armpits or groin that may also be thickened. This is a skin problem called **acanthosis nigricans** – often seen in those with insulin resistance and most common in people with black or brown skin.

Hard, thickened skin on the fingers, toes, or both, is known as **digital sclerosis**. This presents as tight, waxy skin on the backs of your hands and, as a result, your fingers may become stiff and difficult to move. If high blood glucose levels have remained untreated for some time, this can feel like you have pebbles in your fingertips.

Digital sclerosis can spread, with hard, thickened skin having a swollen appearance on the forearms and upper arms. It can also develop on the upper back, shoulders and neck. Occasionally, this skin condition spreads to the face and chest. In rare cases, the skin over the knees, ankles or elbows also thickens, making it difficult to straighten your leg, point your foot or bend your arm. Wherever it appears, the thickened skin often has the texture of orange peel.

Yellowish, scaly patches (known as **xanthelasma**) may develop on or around your eyelids. These are a sign that you have high levels of fat in your blood and can also indicate that you have high blood glucose levels and poor circulation. Reduce the sugar and saturated fat in your diet to remove the yellow areas, and speak to your doctor about having your blood fats and blood glucose measured to check for elevated glucose and high cholesterol levels.

A skin condition called **eruptive xanthoma** causes benign lesions consisting of fatty acid deposits to appear on the skin. They are uncommon and can appear alongside other health conditions. As a result, they may be an early warning sign of another illness that affects the metabolism, such as prediabetes or type 2 diabetes. As with each complication I've described, make lifestyle changes wherever possible to tackle these issues (*see* Part II).

✶ Key messages ✶

- A long-term increase in blood glucose levels is accompanied by a number of complications or secondary health conditions that occur due to cell damage and degeneration.

- Even when it is advanced, damage to the eyes due to high glucose doesn't always cause major sight loss.

- High blood glucose levels can damage blood vessels and nephrons in the kidneys, so they don't work as well as they should.

- Nerve damage, known as neuropathy, can be the first sign of long-term high glucose levels.

- Over time, even slightly raised glucose levels can start to damage blood vessels, which ultimately, in combination with raised cholesterol, can lead to atherosclerosis, the most common cause of a heart attack.

Part II

Actioning change

Chapter 6

Mindset changes

> This chapter helps you break old habits and adopt new ones by altering your mindset with a six-stage behaviour change process.

Making a lasting commitment to behaviour change is not a simple process. It requires time and effort, but even deciding to make a change to your lifestyle is not just a straight progression from decision to action, as you may go backwards as well as forwards. Clearly, to begin the process of change you have to feel ready and be willing to do things differently, but whether you want to lose weight, start a regular exercise programme or reach another health-related target, it may take some time to discover what works best for you. For example, it may not suit you to exercise first thing in the morning, because you're too busy getting the children off to school before you start work, but during your lunch break might be an ideal time.

Behaviour is influenced by many factors and lifestyle change is brought about by modifying at least one of these factors. To be able to start thinking about lifestyle change, you need to feel capable, have the opportunity for change and feel motivated enough to make and sustain change. Most people go through six stages when making and implementing a successful lifestyle change. These stages apply to changing a number of health behaviours, such as healthy eating and weight loss, incorporating regular exercise, improving sleep patterns and stopping smoking, but if you decide to follow them – and I would really encourage you to – you will find they will help you reach your goal.

Beginning the process of change

At first it's all too easy to feel disheartened by the whole idea of trying to do things differently. It's always easier to carry on doing things in the same way, because that doesn't require any extra effort, but even if you are highly motivated, you may be short on time or family support and those things are important, too. The key is to think of ways to change that are achievable and to work out how you can make them manageable. For example, tasks are easier when you divide them up into smaller parts, so when exercising perhaps you could do three 10-minute bursts rather than a constant 30 minutes. Could you walk instead of driving the children to school? Or could you use an exercise bike in front of the TV in the evening and begin a routine in that way?

The things we need to change tend to be unhealthy – like cutting down on fatty, sugary, calorific foods, alcohol or nicotine – but these things give us a boost and make us feel good for a while, which tempts us to consume them again in order to keep experiencing this effect. Eating something with a lot of fat and/or sugar – with the associated endorphin release – is comforting in times of stress or upset, as is drinking alcohol and smoking. Sugar triggers an **endorphin** 'hit' in the brain (hormones such as **dopamine** are released to help relieve stress and provide a sense of wellbeing), making us crave even more sugar, which can then become addictive. However, the same endorphin hit is true of exercise, which is far better for you!

To begin the process of change, you must identify the behaviour you want to change, and recognise its triggers and consequences. For example, perhaps you want to eat in a healthy way, but stress and feeling tired after work mean you eat unhealthy takeaway food instead, feeling guilt, shame, frustration and failure as a result, in addition to gaining weight. It can be a scary process, but don't panic! Working through the stages of change one by one will give you a structure that helps you break old habits and begin new ones by changing your mindset (for more on how to make physical changes, see chapter 7).

> **TIP**
>
> The key to staying on the right track is to recognise why the habit started in the first place. As we have already seen, sugary and fatty foods provide comfort and make us feel happy, as do substances that relax us, like alcohol and nicotine. Recognising that unhealthy habits may stem from life and relationship issues, or your own self-esteem, is a breakthrough moment. Losing weight and reducing your chance of developing prediabetes and type 2 diabetes can help to control these issues. So you can keep track of your successes and the reasons for any relapses – and those reasons could be practical or emotional – it can be helpful to keep a behaviour change diary. Why not start one now?

HOW TO CREATE A BEHAVIOUR CHANGE DIARY

You can start your diary by buying a nice notebook or, if you don't want to carry one with you, you could create the diary on your phone. Design it with simple columns that you can write short notes in:

1. Begin by defining the behaviour you want to change, such as 'I want to do more exercise,' and set some achievable, precise goals, such as 'I will walk for 15 minutes each day.'

2. Write down your As, Bs and Cs:

   A = Antecedent or what happened before. If exercise is your goal, when you think, 'I really should do some exercise this morning,' write down what triggers this thought.

   B = Behaviour or what you did next, after you had this thought. Where were you when you wanted to exercise? Who was present? Was there a particular situation that sparked thoughts of exercising?

   C = Consequence or how you felt.

3. Write down the details. This can be anything that seems relevant, important and potentially helpful. For example, you might want to make a note of:

   - What time you started exercising.
   - How long you exercised for.
   - Whether you feel you are making some progress towards your behaviour change.
   - How often, over the course of perhaps a week, you achieve your exercise goal.

Read through your entries regularly and see if you can spot any barriers to exercising for 15 minutes a day. Was there anything that made exercising harder or easier on certain days? Think of ways to manage any barriers that stop you achieving your goal, so you can keep up the good work. Share your goals with family and friends so that they can give you support.

Behaviour	Goals	ABC	Details
I want to do more exercise	I will walk for 15 minutes each day	**A**ntecedent: I want to stop getting out of breath so quickly **B**ehaviour: I asked my friend to join me and we chose a flat route **C**onsequence: It made me feel good all day so I want to keep going every day, even a little longer	– Days of exercise this week: six – Increased to 20 minutes every other day

Behaviour change is a process, not an event, and you will go through distinct stages of readiness to change. This process acknowledges that you may not necessarily be ready or willing to change, and it recognises that different levels of support are needed at each stage of the journey. These are the six states of readiness for behaviour change:

1. **Pre-contemplation**
2. **Contemplation**
3. **Planning**
4. **Action**
5. **Maintenance**
6. **Relapse.**

❝ **ZOE SAYS:** *I have a few chronic health issues, and this means I have to go to various clinic appointments and check-ups every few months. I know what I'm being told is for my own good, and I do my best to juggle blood glucose with* *type 2 diabetes, high blood pressure, cholesterol levels, exercise and eating healthily. I often feel intimidated by doctors and nurses who always seem to imply that I could be doing more. I won't give up what I'm already doing, but their expectations are rather overwhelming.*

TIP

If you feel intimidated by the expectation that you will automatically want to, or that you should, make changes to your health status, remember that you can only do your best. This also goes for the pressure you put upon yourself by saying, 'I should be doing more exercise' and so on. Don't be too hard on yourself and be realistic about your goals.

Each stage is described below. Read each one through to identify your current readiness for change. As your mindset alters and you commit to changing your lifestyle, read each one through again, and use your behaviour change diary to chart your progress and readiness for change:

Pre-contemplation

This stage describes the time before you become aware of a threat to your health and begin to consider any form of lifestyle change. You may already be aware of an unhealthy behaviour, such as eating too much fat or sugar, taking infrequent exercise or knowing that prediabetes and type 2 diabetes are risks to your health, but you don't yet think of the unhealthy behaviour as something you need to worry about or act upon.

STEVE SAYS: *When I was 34 I was in hospital with a badly broken leg, and they said I had high sugar levels and prediabetes. A diabetes nurse visited me, and she explained the risks and what this meant. It all felt like such a big deal, as though*

> *it wasn't really happening to me. I was worried and anxious, and found it really hard to get my head around it. I suppose it was hard to even think about making an effort to improve my health because I didn't feel ill.*

At this stage you may not be aware that you want – want not should, because the decision must come from you – to make some kind of change, but there will be a trigger. Assessing your prediabetes or type 2 diabetes risk might make you rethink your current behaviours, or an advert on TV or a conversation with friends, family or a health professional about a health subject might have made you view things in a different way. You'll find questions that will help you reflect on what you're doing throughout this chapter.

- Do you see any of your current health behaviours as problematic?
- Are you aware of any negative consequences to your current health behaviours?
- Do you feel you have any control over unhealthy behaviours like not exercising?
- Do you tend to focus on the costs or downside of changing a health behaviour?
- Do you resist making healthy changes, or deny they would be beneficial?
- What would make you change your mind about doing more to improve your health?
- What do you imagine your health status will be in five years? Will you be the same weight?
- If you were told tomorrow that you are at high risk of developing prediabetes or type 2 diabetes, would this act as a trigger for you to consider making a lifestyle change?

Contemplation

Keep calm and take control! Changing behaviour takes a long time, and you are not expected to suddenly be a model person who can snap their fingers and never touch a biscuit again. Choosing healthier food options and being more active can reduce diabetes risk considerably. The most important change must happen from the inside. To be healthier you have to want to lose weight and do more exercise, but focus on your health, not your size.

Contemplation describes your awareness of the benefits of change. At this stage you will consider introducing risk-reducing strategies into your lifestyle and think about how you could sustain these strategies going forward. You may, for example, have recently become aware of the benefits of weight loss or exercise to prevent, manage or reverse prediabetes and type 2 diabetes, and that prompts you to think in more depth about how you could achieve lifestyle changes.

You may think about taking action for weeks or months before you finally feel you can take the next step, but once you recognise the pros and cons of changing a particular behaviour and can identify any potential obstacles that could make changing a behaviour more difficult, you will be ready to do it.

- Have you ever considered the pros and cons of the health behaviour you'd like to change?

- Have you sought out information about changing this behaviour – for example, how to stop smoking?

- Do you have the motivation to change this behaviour and have you acquired some behavioural skills to help you achieve this behaviour?

- What made you realise that you have an unhealthy relationship with food, cigarettes, alcohol or exercise?

- If you have changed that health-related behaviour in the past, how did it go?

- If you were diagnosed with prediabetes or type 2 diabetes tomorrow, would that be enough to recognise that this particular behaviour is a problem?

Getting yourself ready for a lifestyle change – be it dietary, related to exercising more or giving up smoking – requires you to be in the right mindset. It is practically impossible to suddenly alter ingrained behaviours that you may have been doing for many years without some thought and planning. The decision to change a behaviour requires a trigger that makes you realise you want to do things differently and have the motivation to act on that trigger.

> **FAHEEN SAYS:** *I knew I was at risk from type 2 diabetes for genetic reasons, as many of my close family members have it, although I'm not overweight and I wasn't eating unhealthy foods. The news that I'm at high risk was unexpected at my age, as I'm only 36. At a routine health check the nurse suggested I could do more exercise, and eat less salt and fat, with the genetic likelihood of future diabetes in mind. It was hard to get myself to a place where I made more effort to prevent diabetes, because I didn't have any symptoms and felt well. Knowing I was at high risk had niggled away at me for years and I thought about what to do for a long time. Eventually, I realised it was important to get more information, so I did an internet search about prediabetes and learned all I could that way. I also had a chat with the nurse at the doctor's about lifestyle changes I could make. That helped because the general information on the internet then became specific to my own situation.*

If you are diagnosed with prediabetes or type 2 diabetes, though, it will have an instant effect on health professionals as they will leap into action to teach you to manage your condition, even if you're not quite ready for it. You will be asked to attend an intensive in-person or online diabetes education course that is designed to get you to change your lifestyle and behaviour, and you may also be prescribed glucose-lowering medication, although of course it's better to prevent or control prediabetes or type 2 diabetes in the first place, rather than having to manage unstable glucose levels once you have an established health condition.

Of course, if you don't have a diagnosis of prediabetes or type 2 diabetes, have no symptoms and don't feel particularly at risk, you may not feel that you have to do anything at all. Sometimes it is only when a serious threat to your health occurs, like a diagnosis or a heart attack, that you feel the need for change to prevent further ill health, but perhaps you can achieve a state where you're ready to make the change without the threat?

- Why do you really want to change? Be honest with yourself about this.
- What is stopping you from making that change?
- What would help make this process easier and how much can you realistically achieve?

You could begin by gathering as much information about the health behaviour you want to change as possible. For example, if you want to quit smoking, your doctor's practice will provide help and support, with useful information and advice that is tailored specifically to your situation. Looking online for tips on how to quit may also be helpful in providing more generalised advice.

- If you lack motivation and constantly make excuses for not exercising, try not to see the contemplation of a lifestyle change as giving something up, but rather as gaining physically, mentally and emotionally.
- In your behaviour change diary, write down how you could begin to start improving your health. This might include getting some leaflets from your doctor or chemist or identifying sources of support for contemplating a change in your health behaviour.
- In your diary, list what makes change possible for you. This might include family support, strong personal motivation and mindset, your knowledge of the subject, having some free time when you could arrange to do an exercise or yoga class, and so on.

Planning

When you decide to change your lifestyle, diet comes first. This is because what you eat and drink directly influences brain function and behaviour – think of the sugar rush following a high-sugar dessert or the way you feel tired after drinking alcohol. A healthy diet provides the brain with essential nutrients that allow clear thinking, enable decision-making and regulate your mood. Planning what to eat and acting on that plan, though, can feel like the most overwhelming challenge. Because everyone is different and certain things work for some people but not others, there is not one single food plan that will help lower your blood glucose levels. Each person will have their own specific goals that they want to achieve and a way of adapting their lifestyle accordingly (for resources to help you with this, see the next section of this chapter).

This is the time when you decide that making a lifestyle change of any kind is both possible and worthwhile. You may have thought about losing weight and exercising more for a long while, but the time wasn't right. You might now feel ready for a change to occur and you may begin looking at ways to make it happen. This could be a visit to your doctor to discuss weight loss, buying an exercise bike, or asking a friend or family member to join an exercise class with you. You could be in the supermarket and decide not to buy biscuits and crisps so they are not a temptation in the cupboard. Whatever it is, you are planning to do things differently.

When you are planning a behaviour change, be specific about your goals. Instead of aiming to be healthier to prevent prediabetes and type 2 diabetes, set a measurable goal like exercising for 30 minutes, three times a week.

Identify whether your motivation is internal or external motivation. Internal motivation is your own will and desire to achieve your goal, because it is a target you have set yourself, because you realise the benefits to your health and wellbeing. External motivation is when a health professional suggests you should lose weight and exercise more, or quit smoking to improve your health, but the desire to do so does not originate from you. Internal motivation is more sustainable than changing something because someone else wants you to.

Connect your behaviour change to your core values. This means recognising that you want to lose weight and exercise more to prevent, manage or delay the onset of prediabetes and type 2 diabetes for the benefit of your health.

Break down your goal into smaller, achievable steps to avoid feeling overwhelmed. For example, if you have weight to lose, aim to shed one pound a week. Let's say you want to reduce your sugar intake:

- **Your goal**: to reduce sugar consumption by 25% in the next month.
- **Take small steps**: gradually reduce sugary drinks, replace desserts with fruit and carefully read food labels.
- **Get support**: join an online group or read my book for people reducing sugar intake (see p. 178).
- **Coping strategy**: when you have sugar cravings, eat a piece of fruit or go for a walk.
- **Record**: keep a food diary to record your sugar intake.
- **Celebrate**: mark reaching a milestone, like reducing your sugar intake by 10%.
- Why do you engage in your current behaviour? Is it stress, habit or a lack of knowledge?
- What situations or cues led to the behaviour you want to change?
- How will you make your behaviour change happen?
- Are you motivated to change the unhealthy behaviour?
- Who will you approach for help, advice and support to do this?
- Are there any available resources or social support? Would this involve potential barriers such as using public transport or having to rely on someone for a lift?
- What are the benefits to changing this health behaviour?

Activity

In your behaviour change diary (see pp. 76–8), review your goal. Monitor your health behaviour and the outcome – such as walking for 15 minutes each day, and feeling fitter, stronger and more energised for it. If you faced any barriers to carrying out your intention, how did you cope and overcome them? For example, fitting the walk in later in the day or incorporating it with another task, like visiting the library or posting a letter. How will you create your support system – perhaps walk the dog, or walk and chat with a friend or neighbour?

- Make a list of your goals and prepare a plan of how you aim to achieve these milestones. Start experimenting with small, manageable changes.

- Collect some motivational statements and stick them on the fridge so you will see them regularly. A good one to get you started is: 'The greatest discovery of all time is that a person can change their future by merely changing their attitude' (Oprah Winfrey).

❛ **DANNY SAYS:** *I had a lot to change in my life and when I reached 40, I decided it was time to lose weight and quit smoking. I was told by my doctor not to attempt both of these at the same time, but in preparation I started eating lower-fat foods, reducing my portion sizes by one-third and cutting down from 30 cigarettes a day to 20. It's going OK, but I've still got a long way to go. I tell myself that as long as I'm making gradual improvements to my health it doesn't matter how long it takes, but I won't take my eye off the ball. Now I'm planning to cut the cigarettes down to 10 a day as my next goal.* ❜

If you feel like Danny, you will increase your chances of success with a lifestyle change if you gain as much information as possible. Online resources can be good, but make sure they are from reliable sources such as the NHS website, Diabetes UK, the American Diabetes Association or the British Heart Foundation. Get as much support as you can for making your lifestyle change from friends, family, support groups and health professionals.

Action

I know taking action is a big step, and that it's not always easy to make changes to your mindset and lifestyle. However, making a change will have a positive impact on your health, your blood glucose, blood pressure, blood cholesterol levels, positivity and mindset.

When you are in the right mindset to take action, you have made a sustainable decision to do things differently with an achievable goal, realistic plan and support. You will have decided what to change and how you are going to change it. You may have started to cut out certain unhealthy foods and begun moving around more. You may have accommodated exercise into your daily routine or made the decision to reduce your portion sizes – anything that acts on your decision to live a healthier lifestyle. At this stage you have made a commitment to do things differently. When you are ready to take action to adopt behaviour change into your life:

- **Modify your environment**: Support your behaviour change by, for example, removing high-fat, high-sugar foods from your fridge and cupboards to avoid temptation. Ask for feedback from trusted sources who will provide constructive criticism.

- **Find support**: Enlist friends, family and health professionals to help you make and sustain your change. This will boost your self-esteem and confidence and feed back into your efforts, giving you the motivation to continue until you reach your goal.

- **Anticipate**: Think through how you will cope with potential challenges to the change you have made and decide on ways to overcome these issues. For example, if you are attending an event where there will be unhealthy food available, anticipate this and take your own healthier snacks along.

Activity

Create an action plan showing the specific steps you will take to achieve your goal, such as 'I will make my lunch the night before so I won't be tempted to buy something unhealthy in my lunch break.' In this way you are replacing unhealthy behaviours with healthy ones. Monitor your progress so you can see at a glance what is working and where some adjustments might be needed.

- In your behaviour change diary, write down some small, achievable changes you can make to put your plans into action. These could be walking up and down stairs several more times a day or not going on the internet before bed so your mind is relaxed and ready for sleep.

- Don't attempt to make multiple changes at once and give yourself time to get used to doing things differently. Too much too soon won't work. Just try to change one thing at a time and make small, achievable differences.

- Search out people who can help you implement your change: your doctor or other medical professionals, friends, family, support groups, useful books and so on.

- Check in regularly with a friend or family member, perhaps someone who is also trying to change their mindset and adopt a healthier lifestyle. This provides accountability and support.

- No matter how small, celebrate your successes and be proud of yourself. This reinforces positive behaviour.

Opportunity, in the context of behaviour change, refers to external factors that make being able to undertake the behaviour possible. Physical opportunity, opportunities provided by your environment and social opportunity are all part of this. For example, to create the opportunity to begin new dietary patterns, nutrition classes might help. Again, having support from friends or relatives who might also want to join in is a great boost to going ahead with a behavioural decision.

AMARI SAYS: *I didn't really know where to start to make changes, so I looked at what I was unhappy with. My lifestyle had been erratic for a long time and I knew I was the only one who could change it. It sounds strange, but I viewed myself like an outsider looking in, critical of my eating unhealthy things at all hours with no regular routine or concern about nutrition, and drinking when I felt stressed. I was also what is called a 'social smoker'. I would smoke at a party if offered a cigarette, then hate what I'd done afterwards. Things had to change. I made a conscious effort to shop for healthy things* *that I actually enjoyed eating, rather than stuff that I would never touch, making sure I had a proper meal at a regular time, and I stopped snacking during the night. It was a very long and gradual process of really being mindful and thinking about what I was doing, weeding out the rubbish foods, so I wasn't giving everything up in one go. I still don't consider that I'm entirely there yet, but the other day I was offered a cigarette by a friend and I was mindful of wanting to change, so I refused. I didn't miss it and I'm glad I made this decision. It felt like another small step to a better me.*

Get as much social support for making the change as possible. For example, you may want to join a slimming club rather than going it alone, so that you can meet others who want to change the same health behaviour. Social support is very helpful during this time, because behaviour change decisions can fail at this stage, particularly if you haven't spent enough time at the previous stage, and embracing social support is a direct action towards your goal.

KIERON SAYS: *At first I worried about telling people I was trying to lose weight, because I've failed in the past – I didn't want the embarrassment of failing again if people knew – but when I found out I had prediabetes this was my opportunity, making me more motivated than ever to succeed and prevent things from getting worse. In the end I told my family, friends and some trusted work colleagues, and they've been great. With their support and encouragement, I've lost nearly two stone so far and I'll get to my goal of losing three.*

Maintenance

The maintenance stage describes sustained change, usually for longer than six months. At the beginning this may seem like a huge and insurmountable obstacle, but when you get there you will feel empowered to carry on with your good work, with boosted motivation to continue your behaviour change. You will aim to avoid temptation and the possibility of returning to an old behaviour by keeping up the behaviour change you have adopted. The resolve to keep doing the new behaviour is strengthened and you feel confident that you can continue this as a permanent lifestyle change. This may be anything from exercising regularly, not smoking or avoiding alcohol to swerving biscuits, crisps, chocolate and chips.

> **JUDY SAYS:** *It's been very hard to avoid going back to my old patterns of eating, because it's impossible to avoid food. Unlike smoking, eating is necessary for life and food is everywhere – the centre of every occasion. I was eating a plateful of food the same size as my husband was eating and that had to stop. I'm now trying to replace food temptations with exercise and, where possible, a non-food treat. When I want something "nice" to eat after my evening meal, I jog up and down the hallway for 20 minutes. I then feel pleased with myself for not giving in and reward myself with a manicure or pedicure, or a lovely bubble bath. I'm not saying it's easy, but you have to stop focusing on food all the time.*

If you feel like Judy, it's important to use coping strategies to avoid giving in to temptation. To distract yourself from the thought of, say, snacking, regularly remind yourself of your goals and the reasons why you want to change. Rewarding yourself is a way of positively reinforcing the healthy behaviour you have undertaken. This helps to prevent a lapse back to unhealthier patterns of behaviour, such as eating sugary, calorific foods, drinking alcohol or smoking.

One important point is portion sizes. It's all too easy to fill your cereal bowl to the top rather than follow the recommended portion size, which is much less, meaning you are eating far more added sugars. This also goes for eating a quantity of anything that comes in a pre-packed size, like a family bag of crisps, where a portion is one-eighth of a bag. Try cutting your portion sizes down. If it's on your plate (or in the packet), you're more likely to eat it, rather than stopping when you're actually full.

Activity

Stick to consistent routines regarding when you eat and when you exercise, and set a regular bedtime. Establish mindfulness to encourage mental wellbeing, perhaps by practising yoga, if you're physically able. Remember that making a significant change to your health behaviour takes time, so be patient with yourself!

- Consider what it means to make your lifestyle changes permanent.
- Reaffirm your goals and the reasons why you want to change.
- Plan ahead to integrate the new behaviour into your daily routine.
- Make a list of the physical, mental and social benefits that this will bring you in your behaviour change diary.
- Manage your stress to maintain a feeling of control over your intentional change.

Relapse

It's very possible that there will be times when you relapse and return to old habits. This is normal human behaviour, particularly when, for example, you have a stressful day and that threatens your resolve to continue with the change. As you will have seen, reducing high blood glucose levels involves motivation, because you need to make changes to your diet and how frequently you exercise. Having noticed the benefits, some people will be able to keep eating a healthy diet and exercising regularly, but going back to your old ways after a few months of doing things differently is all too easy.

- What has led to the relapse in your behaviour change? Is it still a barrier to changing your behaviour? Maybe the change required effort or time? Perhaps you have a long-term health issue that causes you pain or you are addicted to sugar or nicotine?

- Are you eating unhealthy foods again because you are addicted to fat, salt and sugar? Junk foods provide pleasure and release the hormone dopamine, so we crave them. Dopamine levels can be increased by reducing saturated fat intake in your diet, exercising regularly and getting enough sleep.

- Have you tried to change your lifestyle before, but were unable to maintain your good intentions? Has that had an impact on this relapse?

- Why give up on your lifestyle change plans once you've maintained the behaviour for several months? Changing a long-established habit is difficult and there are often reasons behind these habits that make them easy to return to. Did you have the right mindset?

Barriers to change, or starting again after a relapse, may seem challenging, but there are ways around these issues:

- **Use motivational techniques**: For example, set yourself a bigger goal with small milestones along the way.

- **Do your research and get support**: For example, take up swimming, which will support your body in the water and help with pain, wean yourself slowly off sugar or get help from your doctor to stop smoking.

- **Look for healthier versions of favourite foods**: Identify the products in your fridge, freezer and cupboards that are high in salt, saturated fat and/or sugar, and when you shop, buy similar items that are healthier.

- **Keep up your diary**: Even if you have a relapse, it's worth continuing to keep notes to help you identify cravings, their triggers and how you feel after eating these foods, both physically and mentally.

- **Combat boredom**: Are you eating because you're hungry or because you're bored or fed up? Chewing sugar-free gum or regularly sipping water can suppress the desire to snack, and being mindful of your mood when you want to eat junk food can help you control cravings.

- **Take a measured approach**: Eating balanced meals, taking regular exercise and sleeping well will help you beat junk food addiction.

Embracing the challenge

Habits have been there for a long time and they have become automatic behaviours, so don't expect to change them quickly. Be prepared to deal with a challenge to your chosen behaviour change. Know what might tempt you back into old ways and think of a strategy to avoid this, such as rewarding yourself with a non-food treat. It is common to relapse to previous behaviour patterns, and this can be very disappointing and frustrating. The key is not to let any kind of relapse undermine your confidence that you can achieve your goal. If you do revert to old habits the best thing to do is return to the planning, action or maintenance stages in the behaviour change process.

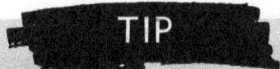

Don't be too hard on yourself if you do take a backwards step, because relapse is a common part of making a significant lifestyle change.

We are all human and it is normal to find maintaining a lifestyle change difficult at times. If you do relapse, identify what triggered it, and reaffirm your target and commitment to change. Reassess your resources and approach, and reassert your plan of action and commitment to achieving the change. Decide how you will deal with any temptation or situations that might deter you in the future.

Habits are formed over many years for a variety of reasons. If you can maintain healthy behaviour change(s), such as healthier eating and regular exercise for six weeks, it is likely that you will be in the right mindset to continue and not look back. These new patterns of healthy behaviour take, on average, nine months to become something you automatically do without having to think about it. If you have maintained healthy behaviours for the milestone nine months you are unlikely to return to your old ways.

However, if you do have a relapse, it is important to realise that this is not the end of the world. You can return to your behaviour change when you feel ready and you will have had the health benefit of the time you were able to enforce the change in your lifestyle.

> **PAUL SAYS:** *I never really linked my overeating and lack of interest in exercising to how I felt about myself. I started to lose weight because my doctor warned that I was on the right path to heart disease and type 2 diabetes. This made me realise that I had mistreated my body for years, because I didn't care enough about myself. Long story short – I'd gone through a messy divorce, lost my home and had no one in my life, so I ate and drank what I liked because it made me feel better emotionally, although not physically. It sounds simple, but understanding the reason why I ate so many unhealthy foods and never exercised changed my outlook to take better care of myself and prevent future ill health.*

Changing what you eat and how you move around can be challenging. Clearly define the behaviour you want to change, whether it's a habit you want to break or a new one you want to form. Understand the context: when, where and why does this behaviour occur? Consider the triggers and consequences of the behaviour.

Define specific, measurable, achievable, relevant and time-bound (SMART) goals. Break down larger goals into smaller, manageable steps. For example, instead of 'lose weight', try 'lose one pound per week by exercising for 30 minutes, three times a week'. Identify strategies that will help you achieve your goals. Consider environmental changes. For example, you could remove unhealthy snacks from your home.

Think about social support. For example, tell a friend about your goals and ask for encouragement or develop a plan to address potential challenges.

Take action by putting your plan into practice. Track your progress and make adjustments as needed. Celebrate your successes along the way. If you're struggling, consider seeking support from a therapist, counsellor or support group. Share your goals with others and ask for encouragement. By following these steps, you can create a solid foundation for successful behaviour change.

> **FACT: It takes, on average, 66 days to change a habit. That means it takes over two months for a new behaviour to become something you do automatically and then nine months for it to really take hold. This does depend on the individual, the behaviour and the circumstances, but change is very much achievable if you stick at it!**

✶ Key messages ✶

- Realising that you could develop prediabetes or type 2 diabetes is the first step towards taking control of your future health.

- Following the six-stage behaviour change process will help you successfully change your behaviour, but it is normal to move backwards as well as forwards through the process.

- Making healthy changes to your diet and being more physically active can reduce the risk of developing prediabetes and type 2 diabetes considerably, with significant benefits to heart health.

- Taking steps to make changes will also benefit your overall health, such as your heart and circulatory system, so even a small change will make a big difference.

- It is important to note that some people do not develop prediabetes or type 2 diabetes because of unhealthy lifestyle choices. It can sometimes be due to a genetic predisposition, ethnicity or linked to certain prescribed medicines.

Chapter 7

Physical changes

> This chapter discusses the range of ways you can make changes to positively affect your diabetes status, from improving your diet and exercising regularly in order to lose weight – including the pros and cons of weight-loss drugs – through to giving up smoking and making sure you attend medical appointments.

Fortunately, there are lifestyle changes you can make to reduce the likelihood of developing prediabetes or type 2 diabetes and, if you already have either of these conditions, you can significantly improve your health. By taking action, it is possible to keep blood glucose within healthy limits and prevent, reverse or improve the management of prediabetes or type 2 diabetes. If you don't make changes, factors you can't control, such as ageing, mean prediabetes and type 2 diabetes may be more likely.

While having consistently high blood glucose levels and being diagnosed with prediabetes is definitely a warning to take care of your health, you won't automatically develop type 2 diabetes – unless you ignore the signs. There is certainly a great deal you can do to prevent prediabetes turning into type 2 diabetes and to avoid developing prediabetes in the first place. What's more, if you already have type 2 diabetes there is also a great deal you can do to stop or even reverse its progression. There are five key ways you can tackle prediabetes and type 2 diabetes, and these are described in the following five sections:

1. **Weight loss through diet and exercise**
2. **Reducing blood glucose levels**
3. **Lowering blood pressure and blood cholesterol**
4. **Stopping smoking**
5. **Going to medical appointments.**

It would be extremely difficult to change everything in all these areas at the same time, and the greater the challenge you set yourself, the more likely you are to give up. I suggest you start by focusing on weight loss and taking more exercise, because changes in those areas will have the most significant impact on your overall health, and if you change what you eat and move more, your blood glucose, blood pressure and blood cholesterol levels will begin to normalise, because these factors will also improve with diet and exercise changes. However, if you're a smoker, you might want to start there (and if you don't smoke, even better, as this is one less thing to tackle) or, if you have no issues with attending medical appointments, you may find that section isn't relevant for you. Remember, though, that to improve your physical health you need to modify your daily habits and routines, and understanding the six stages of the behaviour change process will help you do this (for more on this, see chapter 6).

Weight loss through diet and exercise

Weight loss reduces your risk of prediabetes and type 2 diabetes (for more on this, see chapter 3). This section looks at how you can make dietary changes to achieve weight loss and add physical activity for maximum success. You'll find the following questions will help you reflect on what you're doing throughout this chapter.

- Do you want to lose weight to look better or be healthier? (Of course, it's OK to want to achieve both outcomes!)
- Are you going to change your diet or are you going on a diet? Changing your diet is a permanent overall change for better health – reducing sugar, salt, fat and so on – whereas going on a diet is to achieve weight loss in the shorter term.

Although losing weight is easier said than done, in addition to reducing the risk of prediabetes and type 2 diabetes there are many physical and emotional benefits to carrying less body fat, such as making heart disease and certain cancers less likely, and boosting mood and confidence. Even modest weight loss can result in significant benefits, like reducing blood glucose levels, blood pressure and cholesterol, and gaining energy.

The subject of bodyweight can be a sensitive issue and health professionals tend to focus on weight when there is a health problem, but for most of us dietary changes, along with taking regular exercise, are the most important changes we can make. Diet plays the larger role, with studies suggesting this contributes to around 70% of weight-loss success, while exercise accounts for the remaining 30%. You may find these changes difficult to sustain and many people regain any lost weight over time. However, if you are carrying some extra pounds, losing 5% of your bodyweight has a huge impact on your blood pressure and cholesterol levels, and this will improve your overall health.

ASHLEY SAYS: *Discovering I had prediabetes made me angry at myself. I never cared what food I shovelled into my mouth, so it shouldn't have come as a surprise. But I felt as though my body had let me down, and I knew this was a wake-up call to change my ways. I put myself on a low-carb diet and substituted healthy wholegrains for white bread, white flour and white rice. I read every label on every food item in the cupboards and fridge, assessing the sugar content, and throwing out anything that ranked too high. I told myself*

I was serious about avoiding type 2 diabetes and, although I hated throwing food away, it was worth being ruthless to rid the house of unhealthy rubbish. I bought an exercise bike, cycling for 45 minutes every morning. After two months I'd lost 20 pounds and this spurred me on to do more. I aimed to make myself better and I felt the benefits almost immediately. I lost another 20 pounds over the next few months and now feel like a different person. There is no threat of diabetes on the horizon – amazing! – and I have normal blood glucose levels! It's not a temporary diet; it's a complete lifestyle overhaul and a new way of life. I would urge anyone to do the same if they can. You owe it to yourself.

Prediabetes and type 2 can be put into remission by taking action like Ashley did, but you will always have the underlying risk of these conditions. Losing weight and taking regular exercise helps insulin to work properly and therefore acts to control the risk. However, if you gain weight or become less active again, prediabetes and type 2 diabetes can occur or return, because insulin will be unable to do its job properly and your blood glucose levels will begin to rise once more.

Understanding body mass index

An important step you can take yourself, without having to go to your doctor, is to work out if you are overweight for your height. Health professionals use a calculation based on a person's height and body weight to indicate if they are carrying excess weight. To find out if you are overweight using this measurement, you will need to work out your **body mass index** (BMI).

For adults aged 20 and above, a BMI calculation divides a person's height in metres by their weight in kilograms. For example, if you weigh 70kg (around 11 stone) and you are 1.73 metres tall (5 feet, 8 inches), first square your height: 1.73 x 1.73 = 2.99, then divide 70 (weight in kg) by 2.99 (height in metres squared), giving a BMI measurement of 23.41. This is classed as a healthy weight.

To work out your BMI in feet and inches, stones and pounds, you need to either convert your weight and height to metric units or use an equivalent imperial conversion factor, such as multiplying weight in pounds by 703 and then dividing by height in inches squared. There are many online calculators available that can handle this conversion for you.

- If your BMI measurement is between 18.5 and 24.9, this falls in the healthy range for most adults.

- If your BMI measurement is between 25.0 and 29.9, this falls in the overweight range.

- If your BMI measurement is 30.0 or above, this falls in the obese range.

FACT: A BMI measurement of above 25 increases your risk of type 2 diabetes.

As well as knowing your BMI you can also assess your type 2 diabetes risk by measuring your waist size. Fat that is stored around the abdomen – and therefore around the internal organs – is more of a risk than fat stored around the legs. Measure your waist size with a tape measure (don't use your trouser waist size) for an accurate indication of how much fat is stored there:

- If you are a woman, a healthy waist measurement is 80 centimetres (31.5 inches).

- If you are a man, a healthy waist measurement is 94 centimetres (37 inches).

- If you are a South Asian man, you are at a higher risk of type 2 diabetes, so a healthy waist measurement is four centimetres less (90 centimetres/35 inches).

BMI is often considered less reliable for women compared to men, primarily because it doesn't account for differences in body composition, specifically the higher body fat percentage typically found in women. While BMI uses the same formula for both sexes, it doesn't differentiate between muscle mass and fat mass, and women generally have a higher proportion of body fat at the same BMI as men. Muscle weighs much more than fat.

> **Activity**
> - When you're first thinking about losing weight, focus on your overall health and wellbeing rather than solely on appearance. It doesn't matter what you weigh, what really matters is that you are healthy.
> - Get a notebook and write down how you can remove unhealthy foods from your life: cook your own curries rather than buying ready meals or takeaways; make a shopping list and only buy what's on that list for the healthier meals you're going to make; stop eating chocolate as a snack and buy yourself a non-food treat instead.
> - Think about adopting a sustainable, healthy lifestyle that includes a balanced diet and regular physical activity, rather than quick-fix diets. It is important to recognise that your value is not tied to your weight. Doing this also lifts your mood.

People with excess weight, especially those with obesity and morbid obesity (more than 80–100 pounds above the ideal body weight), have a greater likelihood of developing type 2 diabetes because of the excess weight they carry and the impaired action of insulin. A person who is classed as obese or morbidly obese has an increased risk of prediabetes and type 2 diabetes, heart disease, some cancers, osteoarthritis and sleep apnoea, although there are many other health conditions that are also affected by obesity.

> **FACT: Unsurprisingly, unhealthy eating – too much saturated fat, sugar and processed carbohydrates, and not enough dietary fibre, which helps to regulate blood glucose levels – is a major cause of obesity and contributes towards the development of prediabetes and type 2 diabetes.**

❞ DAVID SAYS: *I am 47 and have worked as a graphic designer for a small friendly firm for the last 15 years. Every lunchtime we would have a couple of pints down the pub, where my usual order of chips with curry sauce would always be waiting for* me. In the evenings I would usually eat out of a tin and I would treat myself to a takeaway at least twice a week. Middle-age spread suddenly caught up with me when I hit 40, but as long as I was happy that was all that really counted.

I usually drink coffee at work and over the years I found it was me who was always making it, because I always needed a drink, but as I always found myself going to the loo as well, I thought that there might be something wrong with my prostate. I plucked up the courage to make an appointment with my doctor. He called me 'morbidly obese' and did a finger prick test on me to find out my blood sugar levels. The result was twice what it should be. He explained that due to my weight it was very likely that I was a type 2 diabetic. He handed me a leaflet and told me to make an appointment for the next week.

When I got home, I googled diabetes and looked up type 2. I read that long-term, type 2 diabetes could lead to blindness and amputation – that is if you didn't die of a heart attack first. I went into panic mode. I kicked myself for every fatty food and pint I had consumed over the years. But was it too late? Was I going to die?

I took a week off work and didn't see anyone except the doctor. He confirmed I was type 2 diabetic. My blood test results were back and my HbA1c said that over the last three months my blood was on average 14 (mmol/L). In that moment, as I left the doctor's surgery, I came to the decision that I wouldn't end up like my father, who was overweight and who died of a heart attack some years ago.

I was put on metformin and vowed I would follow the instructions rigorously. I bought a book on how to live well with diabetes. I went shopping and bought things that didn't come *in cans. I cut out fizzy drinks, not that I drank a lot of them, but they often came as part of a meal deal. A can of fizzy drink is about 140 calories and a pint of lager is 200 calories. If you add them up over a year and divide it by 2500 – the number of calories an adult male should consume – you can work out how many days of extra food you are consuming. Mine was 63!*

I cut out my drinking at lunch times and I joined a local rambling group, rather than going down the pub. Though many of our rambles ended up at one, I would only have a half pint and takeaways became less frequent. I invested in bathroom scales and my weight started to come down.

I've started to feel better in myself and, although I am still overweight and diabetic, I am only two-thirds of the man I used to be. My long-term goal is to lose enough weight so that I am no longer diabetic. If I have any advice it's not to give up. Don't feel sorry for yourself, but get mad at diabetes and beat the bugger. If someone set in their ways like me can do it, so can you!

It can be difficult to get started on losing weight by reducing portion sizes while still trying to include certain foods in your diet and avoiding others. Commercial weight-loss plans can provide structure and guidance on exactly what to eat and in what quantity per day, so this may seem like the ideal answer to shedding the pounds. However, meal replacement milkshakes contain a great deal of sugar (some up to 50%), so these are not advisable for people trying to reduce their risk of prediabetes and type 2 diabetes. Additionally, milkshakes and meal replacement bars do not fill you up and are not suitable if you have a lot of weight to lose as you may be missing out on essential dietary nutrients.

Some commercial weight-loss plans are not designed by nutritionists or dieticians and do not come with lifestyle change education or support to help you adopt healthy and sustainable eating patterns. This is essential as any weight lost quickly will not be maintained and the pounds will return again as soon as you go back to eating as you were previously. Fad diets never work as they are not sustainable. What does work are permanent lifestyle changes, where you understand how you can incorporate a healthy diet and regular exercise into your routine to help you achieve your weight-loss goal over time. Always consult your doctor if you are considering weight loss.

ANNE SAYS: *I was diagnosed with prediabetes, but didn't really understand what that meant in terms of what I could and couldn't eat. I decided to start a meal replacement diet to lose weight without consulting my doctor first. I imagined I would lose weight quickly by having the milkshakes for lunch each day and energy bars for snacks. Not long afterwards, I began to feel unwell with headaches and felt really tired all the time, but didn't link this to the diet foods. I read the food labels and realised the meal replacements were loaded with sugar, and had just made my condition a whole lot worse. I saw my doctor and told him what I'd been doing, then immediately threw the diet foods in the bin as I could have had a heart attack – my sugar level was very high when my doctor tested it. I am now taking medicine to manage the sugar, and trying to lose weight properly with exercise and cutting out fatty, sugary foods, like I should have done in the first place.*

There are also emotional consequences to dieting or changing what you eat. If you have 'been good' all week, having a glass of wine or a small treat at the weekend can make you feel guilty, but it's fine to have the occasional treat as long as it's not too big and not too often. Feeling anxious that the rest of the family wants a takeaway meal for dinner may cause conflict, too, if you're trying to cut down on fat and calories. The answer is everything in moderation.

> **HANIFA SAYS:** *You forget that mood often dictates what to eat and when. I realised that when my husband was working in the evenings and my two sons were out with friends, I basically felt abandoned and would turn to food to make me feel better. I have a high risk of diabetes, but my mind urged me to seek out what was in the fridge for comfort. A friend suggested I should write down everything I ate and drank in a notebook. I thought it was a waste of time, but gave it a go anyway. It was a shock to see I was having an evening meal with my children and then a family bag of chocolate snack biscuits and half a tube of crisps while watching TV later, on my own. I don't even remember enjoying them, just stuffing them in my mouth automatically. I've now started knitting instead, so at least I'm keeping my hands busy, doing something creative and not eating what I don't need.*

You may want to eat comfort food when you're upset, or feel as though you may as well eat what you want because your attempts to change your lifestyle seem to have made no difference to your weight or overall health. These setbacks are common to most people trying to lose weight.

- Do you live to eat or eat to live? If you mainly eat for pleasure rather than nutrition and do not have a balanced diet, this leads to weight gain.
- Is the food you eat good food – lean meat, fish, healthy green vegetables, wholegrain cereals and so on?
- Do you often eat high-sugar, high-fat meals and snacks because they taste nice, as a reward to yourself?

- Do you actually savour your meals and enjoy every mouthful or, on reflection, do you look at your empty plate and think 'that didn't fill me up'?
- After you've eaten your main course do you wait for a while before having a dessert or do you immediately have a sweet treat to 'finish off with'? On average, it takes your brain 20 minutes to process signals from your stomach to indicate fullness.

> **FACT: If sugar is listed as one of the first three ingredients on a food label, avoid that food or drink as the product is high in sugar. Studying food labels allows you to make healthy and informed choices, as you can see which foods contain high levels of saturated fat, salt and sugar.**

When starting something new, you may have concerns and some questions. You may worry about doing more exercise if you have not been active in this way for a while. You may have food allergies or intolerances, and need advice about making changes that take this into account. The first port of call is your doctor or the nurse at your local medical centre, who will be able to give you support and information to reduce your risk of prediabetes and type 2, or help you improve your blood glucose levels if you already have prediabetes or type 2 diabetes.

- There may be a weight management group or diabetes prevention course available in your area. Recent figures, however, show that between 30–70% of people have no access to weight management services local to them, but the NHS has weight-loss apps that can support weight management (*see Resources*).
- Your doctor may order some tests to check the amount of glucose in your blood. You will be told where this test can be performed and when you can expect the results. You may be asked to see your doctor again, depending on the result, in case medication is necessary.

- Weight-loss drugs can be prescribed alongside healthy eating, exercise and psychological support.

- Try not to see food as a comfort – change your mindset and practise thinking differently by recording how you feel in your behaviour change diary (for more on this, see chapter 6).

- Write down what you eat and if you have something high in sugar, fat and calories, how you felt before and afterwards. This will let you identify emotional patterns, and help you recognise what you eat, why and when.

Weight-loss drugs

You may have recently heard about a popular weight-loss drug called **Ozempic**. Hailed as a medicine that reverses type 2 diabetes, Ozempic acts to supress appetite and stops you wanting to eat. With less body fat to impair its action, this then allows insulin to work more efficiently. Although Ozempic, which is injected into the abdomen by a medical professional once a week, was originally prescribed solely for the treatment of type 2 diabetes, it can now be prescribed by a doctor for weight loss without diabetes as well. Of course, this book is focused on preventing and managing high blood glucose levels in the long term, rather than losing weight in the short term, and there are some downsides to using this type of drug, with one of the issues being that intense demand for it to help weight loss has outstripped research into any potential side effects.

Ozempic (also known as Semaglutide and Wegovy) is a drug that can help your pancreas to produce more insulin, improving blood glucose levels and the management of type 2 diabetes. Ozempic achieves this by mimicking glucagon-like peptide-1 antagonist, a hormone naturally produced in the gut, which tells the brain when your stomach is full, regulating your appetite. Ozempic and a similar drug, Mounjaro, improve blood glucose levels and reduce hunger by slowing the rate at which your stomach empties.

> **FACT: Ozempic is a way to temporarily manage type 2 diabetes, resulting in a 15% loss in bodyweight (20% with the drug Mounjaro). As with any weight-loss diet, after stopping Ozempic or Mounjaro, you will regain weight, because your calorie intake is no longer reduced due to appetite suppression. When you come off the drug, regain your appetite, eat more and regain your weight, your blood glucose levels rise and so too does your risk of developing prediabetes or type 2 diabetes.**

Ozempic and Mounjaro are long-term treatments for type 2 diabetes and obesity that can be taken for long periods if they are effective and tolerated. However, lifestyle changes remain an effective way of losing weight to prevent, improve and treat prediabetes and type 2.

With Ozempic it usually takes around eight weeks before the effects of appetite suppression result in any significant weight loss. With lifestyle change you can achieve weight loss more quickly than this and improve or reverse prediabetes and type 2 without the use of medicines like Ozempic. While having injections to help weight management rather than healthy eating and regular exercise may sound tempting, this is not a long-term or risk-free solution. Lifestyle changes with healthy eating and regular exercise is a sustainable option with lasting benefits. Make sure you do your research to make an informed choice about what is best for you before taking any diet or weight-loss medicine.

> **FACT: If you have been prescribed insulin to treat your type 2 diabetes you will need to continue this treatment at a reduced dose, as well as having weekly Ozempic injections. Ozempic works to regulate blood glucose and appetite, while insulin reduces blood glucose levels.**

The disadvantages of using Ozempic

There are obvious disadvantages to losing your appetite. Nutrition is not the same as dietary calories, so to avoid malnutrition it is important that your body still receives the protein, vitamins, minerals and fibre it needs for cell maintenance and repair while eating less food to lose weight. Most of us get at least 50% of our daily calories from ultra-processed foods that are calorie rich, but nutrient poor. It is also necessary to stay active to maintain muscle mass, although your instant energy from food is drastically reduced and your body has to convert stored fat into energy. This means that taking Ozempic to dramatically reduce food intake and calories to lose weight is not risk-free.

Taking Ozempic for weight loss and type 2 management can also have digestive system side effects, such as stomach pain, nausea, vomiting and diarrhoea or constipation. These are the most common experiences and some people decide to stop having injections of Ozempic as a consequence. Ozempic has allegedly been associated with severe side effects, such as inflammation of the pancreas (**pancreatitis**), and several deaths: some of the deaths occurred due to severe complications, while others were classed as 'sudden death' attributed to the diabetes drug itself.

❝TERESA SAYS: *I am not overweight, but I was outside the school gates, waiting to pick up my children, when the subject of weight-loss jabs came up. Some of the mums were using the pens (obtained on prescription from a private doctor) and I was offered one. Everyone wants to be a bit thinner, so I am ashamed to say I took it home and injected it into my abdomen just to try it and see what effect it had. That evening I felt really sick and had no appetite. I felt terrible, with low mood and no energy. My husband thought it was a stomach bug, but I didn't tell him what I'd done. I was vomiting constantly and visiting the toilet. This lasted two weeks and I didn't feel normal again for a couple of months. I did lose weight from not eating and having no appetite, but after the drug had left my system I was* *ravenous. A friend who was taking it for several months has now stopped because of the cost and she's put all the weight she lost back on, plus a load more. I really wouldn't advise anyone to take this, because it makes you feel really unwell and the weight doesn't stay off anyway.*

There are other serious side effects to be considered before taking Ozempic for weight loss alone rather than as a prescribed medicine for your type 2 diabetes, including:

- Loss of bone and muscle mass
- Inflammation of the pancreas and destruction of the insulin-producing pancreatic islet cells
- Increased risk of developing sudden loss of vision in one eye, caused by damage to the optic nerve
- Blurred vision – and for those with diabetic retinopathy this can become worse
- Increased risk of impaired kidney function or even kidney failure
- Increased risk of blood glucose levels falling too low (**hypoglycaemia**), especially if you take insulin to manage type 2 diabetes
- Increased risk of developing thyroid cancer and gallbladder disease.

As you can see, there are a number of serious potential side effects associated with taking Ozempic, although your doctor may still prescribe it for the management of type 2 in the short term. If you are concerned about your weight, prediabetes or type 2 diabetes, then speak to your doctor.

> **FACT:** Weight-loss drugs are not a magic bullet that will solve the issue of obesity. That can only be done successfully with lifestyle changes that improve long-term health.

Health benefits of weight loss

As we have seen, excess weight is also associated with reduced insulin sensitivity, increasing the risk of eventual progression to prediabetes and type 2 diabetes or making it harder to manage these conditions. If you already have high blood pressure and type 2 diabetes, these health conditions can be prevented or vastly improved with weight loss. Losing between 5 and 7% of your bodyweight (around 10 to 15 pounds for someone who weighs 200 pounds) improves insulin sensitivity, lowers blood glucose and, in turn, prevents or reverses prediabetes. This also relieves the workload on the insulin-producing cells of the pancreas, preserving their function for longer.

If you are at increased risk or already have prediabetes or type 2 diabetes due to age, genetic factors, ethnicity or prescribed medication you take, it may seem that weight reduction will not be effective in preventing or improving these conditions. Weight loss, however, will enable insulin to work correctly, improving blood glucose levels. Losing weight reduces the risk of developing prediabetes by 58%. If you already have or want to prevent prediabetes or type 2 diabetes because you are at high risk, healthy eating and regular exercise is the way forward. In general, men require 2500 calories a day and women require 2000 calories. To achieve weight loss, men require 1900 calories a day and women require 1400 calories.

DIABETES REVERSAL PROGRAMME

A year-long type 2 diabetes reversal programme run by the NHS found that one-third of participants lost nearly 16kg (35 pounds) putting their type 2 diabetes into remission. Participants ate 900 calories per day, comprising shakes, soups and meal replacement bars, although solid foods were later reintroduced. However, sticking to this regime to prevent type 2 diabetes from returning was challenging. This is why permanent lifestyle change is essential.

The purpose of weight loss and lifestyle change is to help insulin work more effectively to regulate blood glucose levels. This, in turn, reduces the risk factors associated with prediabetes or type 2 diabetes, helping to delay, manage and reverse these conditions. To reduce your risk of prediabetes and type 2 diabetes, there are some simple food choices you can make:

- Avoid full-sugar fizzy drinks and energy drinks, and choose options with no added sugar, including tea and coffee.
- Don't drink fruit juice or smoothies as these contain high levels of fructose – fruit sugar. Fruits such as mango and pineapple have the highest sugar content.
- Avoid white bread, white rice and pasta as these have had their dietary fibre removed.
- Eat wholegrain bread, brown rice and brown pasta to increase the fibre content of your diet. These foods allow a slow release of glucose into the bloodstream rather than causing a sharp increase.
- Eat pulses, such as beans, lentils and chickpeas.
- Eat healthy plant foods, such as tomatoes and peppers, leafy greens, broccoli, cauliflower and whole oats.
- Go for fibre-rich foods, because they are more filling and energy rich, and fibre slows the absorption of glucose in the intestines, which reduces blood glucose levels and has a beneficial effect on how dietary fats and cholesterol are absorbed. Dietary fibre also helps reduce inflammation and blood pressure.
- Choose unsweetened yoghurts. Many low-fat yoghurts are high in sugar because the sugar content makes up for the reduction in fat by giving the product 'mouth feel' and substance.
- Don't eat sugary breakfast cereals. The vast majority of cereals contain a high amount of added sugar. Choose porridge oats or original shredded wheat for a low-sugar/high-fibre breakfast and always read the labels.
- Reduce your intake of processed meats like ham and bacon, which are less heart-healthy and are high in salt. Choose lean chicken

and fish, such as salmon and mackerel, eggs and unsalted nuts as healthier sources of protein. In August, 2024, a study of two million people from 20 countries found that both red and processed meats, like steak, sausages, ham and bacon could increase the risk of developing type 2 diabetes. However, this is dependent on how much and how often these foods are eaten, indicating that a balanced diet is necessary.

- Consume foods that have been found to specifically reduce the risk of type 2. Particularly beneficial are green leafy vegetables, such as spinach, rocket, watercress and kale. Fruits associated with reducing the risk of prediabetes and type 2 diabetes include berries (particularly raspberries), apples and grapes.

- Avoid having alcohol every day, as binge drinking – defined as consuming a large amount of alcohol several times a week – is particularly bad for the health and increases the risk of conditions such as cancer and liver disease. Alcohol is also high in calories and contributes towards being overweight and obesity around the waistline.

- Snack on healthier options, such as pumpkin seeds, unsalted nuts, plain popcorn without sugar, butter or salt, or unsweetened yoghurts, instead of biscuits, cake, crisps and sweets.

- Avoid unhealthy fats, such as butter, lard, ghee, fatty meat, cream, palm oil, coconut milk, cakes, biscuits, pastries and pies. These types of fat are also damaging to the heart and contribute to heart disease. Eat lean meat and use low-fat spreads, and olive, sunflower or rapeseed oil for cooking as an alternative.

- Avoid adding extra salt to food and limit consumption to one teaspoon a day in cooking (it's better not to add it at all). Try adding herbs and spices to cooking to enhance flavour instead of salt. A diet high in salt is associated with high blood pressure, increasing the likelihood of heart disease and stroke, and also increasing the risk of type 2 diabetes and kidney disease.

> **CAROL SAYS:** *I was at my doctor's for something else and I picked up some weight-loss leaflets. After the nurse told me about prediabetes because my sugar levels were slightly raised, I started reading up on healthy diet tips online. I haven't got prediabetes, but I also wanted to lose some weight, so I decided to make changes that the whole family could benefit from. I made it into a game to see if we could eat well for a month. We all stopped having a sugary chocolate cereal for breakfast, replacing it with plain shredded wheat. The kids complained, but I told them it was just to see if we felt better for it. Then we stopped having white bread for packed lunch or toast and tried a seeded loaf instead that everyone agrees is nicer. We had fresh fruit in our lunchboxes, too, instead of a cupcake or chocolate biscuit and crisps. Evening meals were made up of brown rice, wholewheat pasta or a jacket potato, and we had low-sugar sauces on the pasta and lots more vegetables. After four weeks of eating like this, we all felt better physically, had lost some weight, and agreed to continue, because it's really worth it and not actually that difficult.*

In terms of helping insulin work, certain nutrients, such as magnesium, calcium, potassium and dietary fibre, are essential. Many people don't consume enough of these nutrients, resulting in elevated blood glucose levels and insulin resistance. Here is a list of nutrients and dietary supplements that can enable insulin to work more effectively:

- **Alpha-lipoic acid**: A natural **antioxidant** compound, alpha-lipoic acid (ALA) neutralises substances that damage cells, cause illness and ageing. ALA has positive effects on the regulation of insulin sensitivity and insulin secretion, and is widely prescribed for people with nerve damage (diabetic polyneuropathy) and other insulin resistance conditions.
- **Berberine**: Also known as berberine hydrochloride, this is an ingredient in Chinese herbal medicines that can help reduce blood

glucose and has been called 'nature's Ozempic'. It can promote the production of insulin-producing beta cells in the pancreas and in recent years has been widely used in the treatment of type 2 diabetes.

- **Calcium**: Low levels of calcium are associated with impaired glucose metabolism, and insufficient calcium has been associated with high blood pressure and obesity, both of which are factors in insulin resistance. One clinical trial found that calcium supplementation reduced fasting plasma insulin and increased insulin sensitivity in non-diabetic individuals with high blood pressure.

- **Chlorella**: A green algae, rich in chlorophyll, chlorella benefits include lowering blood glucose and it is a good source of protein, fat-soluble vitamins, choline, dietary fibre and essential minerals.

- **Chromium**: Insulin resistance is associated with very low chromium intake and chromium supplements may reduce blood glucose levels, as well as the amount of insulin people with diabetes need. There is some evidence that chromium supplements might reduce food intake, hunger levels and fat cravings, although too much chromium may actually worsen insulin sensitivity.

- **Cinnamon**: Often used in cooking and baking, cinnamon has increasingly been positively linked with health conditions such as diabetes and cinnamon bark has long been recognised as an aid to reducing blood glucose and cholesterol levels in people with type 2 diabetes.

- **Fish oil supplements**: Associated with a lower risk of metabolic syndrome, fish oil benefits a wide range of chronic health conditions, including type 2 diabetes. Fish oil also increases insulin sensitivity among those with metabolic disorders.

- **Magnesium**: High levels of magnesium have been shown to improve glucose metabolism and stabilise insulin levels. Low levels of magnesium have been associated with elevated blood glucose (hyperglycaemia) and insulin resistance. Additionally, waist circumference is independently associated with low magnesium levels and magnesium supplementation improves insulin sensitivity even in people who are overweight, but don't have diabetes.

- **Potassium**: Low levels are associated with diabetes onset and high dietary potassium intake reduces the risk of insulin resistance.
- **Vitamin C**: In a study examining the effects of vitamin C on blood glucose levels, researchers found that people with type 2 diabetes who took a vitamin C supplement had lower post-meal levels of glucose.
- **Vitamin D**: Researchers found that taking vitamin D_3 (*cholecalciferol*) increased sensitivity to insulin levels and significantly reduced the level of insulin resistance. Vitamin D supplements can help reduce obesity, BMI and waist circumference, although too much vitamin D can have disadvantages for health. Vitamin D toxicity can cause dangerous calcium build-up which can in turn cause issues such as kidney damage and weakened bones.

Taking more exercise

Exercise may be the last thing you want to change, but it is undoubtedly a vital factor in weight control. Being more physically active each day will help you reach and maintain a healthy weight and stabilise your blood glucose levels.

> **FACT: Physical activity is defined as any movement requiring energy expenditure, including occupational work, walking and cycling, household chores, sport and planned exercise. These activities are associated with a 20–30% risk reduction, especially for those at high risk of prediabetes and type 2 diabetes. Increased physical activity is especially beneficial for weight reduction: two and a half hours of brisk walking at a moderate intensity per week reduces diabetes risk by 27%, independent of your body weight. Therefore, it doesn't matter what size you are: increased activity brings substantial health benefits.**

Insulin works more efficiently when your body is active, but you don't have to find time to participate in a particular sport. Activity basically means moving your body. You may feel that you are already fairly active, because you're always on the go, walking to work or around the house, but whatever your current level of activity, aim to increase it. That doesn't necessarily mean taking out a gym membership or jogging around the park every day. It can be bending and flexing your arms and legs while sat watching television.

- Do you often think that you really should do more exercise, but never get around to it?
- What would make it easier for you to exercise more? For example, more time, more motivation, more support?
- If you aim is to do a specific number of exercise sessions per week, is that putting you off? Try to incorporate exercise into your daily routine instead.
- Do you see exercise as a chore? Choose enjoyable activities like dancing or swimming with friends. Do this consistently to make regular activity a habit.
- Have you considered using a fitness tracker to monitor your progress and help you stay motivated?

> **FACT: Regular exercise reduces the risk of developing type 2 diabetes by 40%.**

Excess body fat, especially visceral fat around the organs, can interfere with the ability of insulin to regulate blood glucose levels, leading to insulin resistance – where body cells don't respond effectively to insulin. Insulin resistance can then lead to prediabetes and, if not recognised, diagnosed and managed, eventually type 2 diabetes. Unsurprisingly, there is a strong link between being overweight and taking little or no exercise.

For relaxation, many people tend to choose activities where they are sitting down, such as watching TV, playing computer games or browsing the internet, rather than taking regular physical exercise, but if you're not active enough, you don't use the energy provided by the food you eat and this excess energy you consume is stored by your body as fat. Your metabolism is also sluggish, so insulin works less efficiently to regulate blood glucose levels.

How much exercise should I do?

Knowing how much exercise you should be taking is often confusing. The NHS recommends that adults aged 19–64 engage in some type of daily physical activity, but exercising just once or twice a week can reduce the risk of heart disease and stroke. Government guidelines currently suggest that 150 minutes of moderate exercise each week (30 minutes per day) can reduce diabetes risk, but what exactly is 'moderate' exercise? Exercise intensity over 30 minutes can be defined as low, moderate or vigorous.

- **Low intensity**: Physical activity done at a comfortable pace, such as climbing stairs, shopping, ironing or washing dishes.

- **Moderate intensity**: Physical activity done at least five times a week that makes you feel warmer, and increases your breathing and heart rate, such as digging the garden, pushing a pram, climbing stairs at a pace, walking the dog or washing the car. It doesn't have to be 30 minutes of continuous exercise – it can be several shorter periods of activity totalling 30 minutes a day.

- **Vigorous, sustained exercise**: Physical activity that makes your breathing become hard and fast, and increases your heart rate considerably. Examples of vigorous exercise include jogging, running and cycling. However, intensive exercise can actually increase, rather than lower, blood glucose, because the liver releases more glucose than the exercising muscles need. Always consult your doctor before starting any new physical regime.

Do 150 minutes of moderate intensity physical activity or 75 minutes of vigorous activity weekly. You can mix moderate, intensive and vigorous exercise. The amount of activity can be achieved in one session or spread over several days to reach the required total. Do activities twice a week that improve your muscle strength and spend less time sitting or lying down, so you have fewer long, inactive periods.

If you have decided to walk more as your chosen form of exercise, buying a pedometer is a good way to put your plan into action. If you're not doing them already, measuring the steps you currently do allows you to see how many more you need to do to reach 10,000 a day.

> **FACT: You may not need to lose weight, but you may still be at risk of prediabetes and type 2 diabetes. One of the benefits of being more active is that this will help you reduce this risk.**

Moving more and spending more time being active is a good preventative measure against prediabetes and type 2 diabetes. However, this is easier said than done. You may be unable to undertake certain activities due to health problems such as arthritis or asthma, but as long as you are moving more, even if this is using a mini pedal exerciser while sitting in a chair, this will be beneficial to your blood glucose levels and your overall health.

> **PAM SAYS:** *I hadn't done any serious exercise for many years due to an arthritic knee. With anti-inflammatory tablets I was able to walk without pain, so I've been walking 30 minutes every day for six months now. It was an easy exercise to incorporate into my lifestyle, and I've lost weight (helping my knee with less weight to support) and I now sleep better. My doctor told me that as a person who had been on the borderline of prediabetes for some time, walking has improved my blood glucose levels and how my body uses insulin. He said walking has been as effective as running or doing vigorous exercise in lowering my risk of getting prediabetes and then type 2 diabetes later in life. Walking has also reduced my blood pressure, heart attack and stroke risk.*

Walking is an activity that can easily be made a part of your lifestyle to prevent or reverse prediabetes and type 2 diabetes. Researchers have found that walking for 11 miles over one week (that's just over 1.5 miles a day) acts to reverse prediabetes in the same way as treating prediabetes with dieting. This means that a simple activity like regular walking can have a huge impact on reducing blood glucose levels, reducing prediabetes risk or reversing this condition if you already have it, as well as preventing or vastly improving type 2 diabetes.

You can begin by moving more for 15 to 20 minutes during light physical activity, slowly increasing the length and intensity of the activity over the following weeks. As we have seen, you should aim for between 30 and 60 minutes of moderate exercise five times a week. You can ask your doctor about the NHS Exercise Referral Scheme, typically lasting 12 weeks. Friends and family could join, too, to support and motivate you.

Another key prevention measure, if you are physically able, is getting the large muscles like those in the buttocks and thighs working with high intensity and resistance exercise. This type of activity allows large muscles to take up glucose in the blood to use for fuel, reducing blood glucose levels for 48 hours afterwards. Exercise and a healthy diet go hand in hand to prevent, reverse or improve prediabetes and type 2.

Although it is always good to get fresh air, you don't have to go outside to walk in a park or along a seafront, because you can achieve the same health effect by walking up a set of stairs. This boosts oxygen circulation, helping hormones such as **norepinephrine**, **epinephrine** and cortisol to enhance energy. Stepping up and down on one stair to lift your body from the floor works large muscle groups in your thighs and buttocks that may not be used as much when walking.

Those who succeed in losing weight permanently are the ones who adopt a more active lifestyle. It's not necessary to suddenly begin a strenuous exercise routine – you should start slowly and build up your endurance over time, especially if you have not exercised for a while. This applies if you're pregnant or have a disability, too, but make sure the chosen activity is suitable for your level of physical fitness. Always consult your doctor for advice.

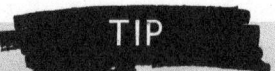

A moderate-intensity exercise level means you should be breathing harder and feeling warmer. You should still have enough breath to talk, but not enough to sing.

Regular activity and weight loss is the best way to help insulin work correctly to reduce blood glucose levels, improve existing prediabetes and type 2, and lower your prediabetes and type 2 diabetes risk. Exercise has an ongoing beneficial effect on glucose levels that can last up to 24 hours.

> **Activity**
> - Decide how you are going to introduce moving more into your lifestyle and write this in your behaviour change diary, charting your progress.
> - Choose an activity you will enjoy and can commit to, like swimming, dancing or walking the dog.
> - In your behavioural change diary or phone planner, schedule exercise sessions like appointments, so you know you've made time for them.
> - As with all lifestyle changes, make the goal realistic.

There is a lot of information in this section, which I hope hasn't been too overwhelming, but it should help you make achievable changes to your food and exercise choices that will in turn reduce your prediabetes and type 2 diabetes risk or, if you have already developed them, enable you to manage these conditions more effectively.

Reducing blood glucose levels

Blood glucose describes the concentration of glucose in your blood. This is your body's primary source of energy and it's derived from the food you eat. However, when glucose levels stay high after meals, it damages the cells in your body, so maintaining healthy blood glucose levels is crucial for overall health, and imbalances can lead to various health issues, including prediabetes and type 2 diabetes.

Many people are not aware of high glucose levels until a health problem occurs (for more on symptoms of prediabetes and type 2 diabetes, *see* chapter 2) and people who have been diagnosed with elevated blood glucose levels are often concerned about what it might mean for the future. There are a number of factors that raise blood glucose, but there are many measures you can take to help bring your blood glucose levels down and thus prevent type 2 diabetes, and any of the other complications of long-term high glucose levels, such as eye, kidney and heart disease, developing. As always, the best way to start is by keeping it simple:

- **Focus on healthy eating**: To lower your blood glucose levels, write down three positive changes you can make to your diet this week – that means more fibre, fewer sugary and starchy foods, and staying hydrated – and work towards making those changes.
- **Increase your physical activity**: As we saw in the last section, you can divide a 30-minute exercise session into three 10-minute sessions, which is a good starting point and will hardly disrupt your usual routine at all.
- **Take advice**: If a health professional has said you have high glucose levels, they will have given you further advice, so do what they say and take any medication they have given you.

The glucose in your blood is mainly derived from the food you eat, but what type of food you eat – for example, whether or not it's a carbohydrate that's quickly converted into glucose – and when you eat it can have a significant impact on your blood glucose levels. Other factors, like stress or medications, can also have an impact. In this section I'm going to take you through these broad categories of food, introduce you to the glycaemic index, and touch on some of those other factors, to give you an understanding of factors that affect your blood glucose levels.

Carbohydrates

Many foods contain simple carbohydrates – sugar molecules – which are quickly converted to glucose to be used by the body as energy, rapidly raising blood glucose and increasing the risk of developing prediabetes and type 2 diabetes. Any glucose not used to keep brain, heart, respiratory and digestive function going, or for physical tasks, is stored in the liver. This triggers the release of insulin, preventing glucose build-up becoming toxic to the brain and body cells.

However, healthy (complex) carbohydrates that include sources of fibre, good fats and protein can help reduce your risk of prediabetes, type 2 diabetes and also heart disease. Any lifestyle change that helps you shed excess weight will also improve your blood glucose and cholesterol levels. There are other advantages to eating a healthy carbohydrate diet containing fibre, such as weight loss without hunger, because higher-fibre foods stay in the stomach for longer, helping blood glucose and blood pressure to return to normal, reducing sugar cravings.

> **FACT: Sugars are the building blocks of all carbohydrates. Sugars are made of single molecules like glucose, fructose (fruit sugars) and galactose (milk sugar), or several molecules that combine to form other sugars, such as sucrose (table sugar). Single-molecule sugars raise blood glucose levels very quickly.**

To dramatically reduce your diabetes risk, you can cut out carbohydrates that quickly become glucose, such as:

- White bread, white pasta, white rice and cereals
- Starchy vegetables like potatoes and sweetcorn
- Biscuits, cake, sweets, jam and honey
- Snacks like crisps and crackers
- Fruits (particularly bananas, mango, pineapple), fruit juices and smoothies
- Milkshakes, sweetened milk products and sweetened soy milk.

> **FACT: Insulin encourages fat storage in the body. Eating carbohydrates like biscuits, cakes and sweets means more insulin is produced to deal with the amount of glucose these foods contain. Any excess glucose in the blood is then stored as fat. In type 2 diabetes, extra insulin is released to process carbohydrates because cells in your body aren't able to use insulin effectively.**

For a diet that helps keep blood glucose levels under control the aim is not to cut out all carbohydrates, but to only eat foods that raise blood glucose slowly. These are higher-fibre foods like wholewheat (brown) pasta, brown rice and porridge oats. There are different types of carbohydrates and it is important to choose what you eat with the knowledge that you are choosing a healthier option.

KAI SAYS: I lowered my type 2 diabetes risk by only eating good carbohydrates. I bought myself a couple of low-carbohydrate cookbooks that contained recipes I knew I'd actually enjoy making and eating, and could afford to buy. I then cut out bread and potatoes, and swapped to brown rice and wholewheat pasta. I cleared my cupboards, fridge and freezer of high-sugar drinks and processed foods – pizzas, pies, sugary desserts, tinned fruit in syrup, tomato sauce and pickle with a high sugar content. With nothing unhealthy in the house, I had no choice but to eat well. It took some getting used to and I had terrible cravings for sugar and junk food for a few weeks, but then it became much easier. Now my blood glucose levels don't spike, so I no longer feel awful after eating and I spend much less time shopping in the supermarket, as there are so many aisles I don't need to go down now.

There are three types of carbohydrate and each of these is converted into energy:

- **Sugars**: These occur naturally in some foods while others are added during manufacture.
- **Starches**: These are a part of most fruits, vegetables and grains.
- **Fibre**: These are the parts of food that are not broken down by the body.

Sugars

In addition to increasing blood glucose levels, sugar of any type has a negative effect on the body. As a substance, the impact of seemingly innocent sugar is as addictive as nicotine, alcohol, morphine or heroin, having similar effects on the brain's reward system, known as the limbic system. Sugar is harmful because it affects chemical messengers in the brain, which can result in an addiction to sugar. A diet that is high in sugar can lead to excess glucose in the blood and this excess, from over-consumption or the body's inability to process glucose in prediabetes and type 2 diabetes, ultimately damages brain structures, causing memory deficiencies.

> **FACT: Naturally occurring sugars in fruit (fructose) and milk (lactose) are not healthier than the range of sugars added to food and drink by manufacturers. Sugar is sugar, wherever it originates from.**

Fruit sugar (fructose) increases the amount of insulin required after a meal in order to reduce blood glucose levels; fruit sugar also increases levels of **adrenocortical hormone** and oestrogen. Adrenocortical hormones are steroid hormones produced by the outer layer of the adrenal glands located on top of the kidneys. The main adrenocortical hormones are cortisol, which regulates stress, metabolism, and inflammation; and the androgens, which contribute to male sex hormone characteristics. An increased level of one hormone in the body has an impact on the body's chemical processes, leading to an imbalance of other hormones.

The hormone **ghrelin** stimulates appetite and hunger, and promotes fat storage. Sugar triggers the release of this hormone and decreases the normal action of another hormone, known as **leptin**, which helps us burn fat for energy when eating a low-carbohydrate diet. This means that the action of sugar on these hormones leads to weight gain. Eating sugar changes how body cells are able to work, making them less able to function normally. This happens in diabetes, where body cells are unable to use glucose as fuel if too much glucose is present in the blood.

Manufacturers tend to pack foods with sugars and fats to make them taste appealing, and sugar is added to savoury foods like burgers, baked beans, soups, pickles and sauces. When foods are labelled as diet options, they tend to be lower in fat, but then have a high sugar content to give the product 'mouth feel'. The high-sugar, high-fat culture we live in – where fast food is instantly available on the high street or via an app – can be blamed for the current obesity crisis.

> **FACT: Sugars added to food by manufacturers, the cook or consumer have no nutritional value. Sugar in any form causes metabolic upset and the development of serious health problems like obesity, heart disease, and prediabetes and type 2 diabetes.**

We crave foods containing sugar because they taste nice, provide a temporary 'high' and are addictive, although this addiction can be beaten. it's impossible to completely avoid all types of sugar unless you grow all your own food and make your own meals from scratch without adding any type of sugar, honey, molasses and so on, but you can cut out all high-sugar manufactured foods like breakfast cereals, yoghurts and sauces. If you look at food packaging you will find there are many different descriptions of sugar in food, such as 'total sugars', 'free sugars' and 'added sugars'.

The latter are extracted or produced from naturally occurring sources, such as the glucose or fructose from fruits, vegetables, honey or milk, and are added to foods in the preparation process. This means that the source of sugar in a biscuit, of low nutritional value, is the same as in a piece of fruit, containing other nutrients and fibre. We are consuming more and more added sugar, because sugar has so many uses in food manufacturing. This increases the extent by which sugar can have a detrimental effect on health. While manufacturers justify the use of sugar in foods because it provides texture, is a flavour enhancer, absorbs water, acts as a preservative, and provides body and mouth feel to foods, the reality is that significant amounts of sugar are now being added to almost all processed foods.

FACT: Current estimates of UK sugar intakes from the National Diet and Nutrition Survey programme show that school-aged children and teenagers are now eating three times more sugar every day than is recommended. Adults are consuming around twice the maximum recommended level of sugar per day.

OTHER NAMES FOR SUGAR

On food labels, sugar is listed under many different names, including:

Agave syrup; barley malt; beet sugar; brown sugar; brown rice sugar; cane sugar; confectioner's sugar; corn syrup; corn sugar; date syrup; dextrin; dextrose; fructooligosaccharides; fructose; fruit juice concentrate; galactose; glucose; granulated sugar; high fructose corn sugar; honey; invert sugar; lactose; maltodextrin; malted barley; maltitol; maltose; mannitol; maple sugar; microcrystalline cellulose; molasses; polydextrose; powdered sugar; raisin juice (fructose); raisin syrup; raw sugar; sorbitol; SUCANAT; sucrose; sugar cane; turbinado sugar; white sugar; xylitol.

Although we are encouraged to eat more fruit, this increases the amount of fruit sugar (fructose) we consume. The guideline of 'five a day' really means that you should eat only two pieces of fruit and three different vegetables each day as a minimum. In other countries the guideline is seven a day – five vegetables and two fruits. Eating a lot of fruit is not a healthy option, and dried fruits like apricots, sultanas, figs, dates and raisins contain high amounts of concentrated sugars, which leads to high blood glucose levels.

> **FACT: As fruit ripens it becomes sweeter, because the glucose contained converts to fructose. The same is true of potatoes. Older potatoes have more carbohydrate because they contain less water, so the carbohydrate is more concentrated. This also goes for French fries. Dried potato, where you add water, is especially high in carbohydrate.**

You might think that snacking on fruit instead of sweet foods would be a healthier option, but, although you may not realise it, eating more than two pieces of fruit a day has a negative effect, because it:

- Increases blood glucose levels
- Increases blood pressure and blood fats
- Encourages the accumulation of body fat around your central organs
- Increases the risk of heart disease
- Creates a build-up of uric acid in the blood causing **gout**, a painful inflammatory arthritis
- Increases cortisol, the stress hormone.

Without a label it is difficult to know exactly how much fruit sugar a piece of fresh fruit contains, although it's easier to determine for tinned fruit in natural juice (never eat tinned fruit in sugar syrup). Vegetables such as beetroot, sweetcorn and carrots contain more fructose than other vegetables, although this is far less than you would find in fruit, so even the sweetest vegetables are equivalent to fruits with a low fructose content.

Sugar is an addictive substance that makes you feel good when you eat it, because it satisfies the brain's pleasure-seeking tendencies. Sugar causes feel-good hormones to be released by the brain, increasing pleasure emotions. Reducing your sugar intake slowly is the best way to remove unnecessary sugar from your life that will increase blood glucose and heighten your risk of prediabetes and type 2 diabetes.

If you are trying to cut down on unhealthy sugars and fats to reduce diabetes risk, you might like to know what amounts are considered healthy and unhealthy. A food is high in sugars if it contains more than 22.5g of total sugars per 100g. It is classed as low in sugars if it contains 5g of total sugars or less per 100g.

Starches

As we have already seen, you can reduce your prediabetes and type 2 diabetes risk with the knowledge that wholegrain bread, brown pasta, potatoes including their skins, rice, high-fibre breakfast cereals, oats and other grains such as rye and barley are starchy foods that provide energy. Although these foods are often referred to as 'carbs', this is not strictly the case as carbohydrates include both starch and sugars, as well as fibre. Starchy foods are also rich in nutrients, providing B vitamins, iron and calcium, so half of your daily calories should come from these carbohydrates.

> **FACT: Eating wholegrain or wholemeal bread, wholewheat pasta and brown rice, and leaving the skins on potatoes provides more fibre. The recommended level of daily fibre is 30g for adults. These starchy carbohydrates should make up one-third of your diet, although in the UK research shows that the average diet contains only one-fifth starchy carbohydrates.**

Starches such as wholegrain bread, wholewheat pasta or potatoes steadily maintain blood glucose levels, so they reduce risk because they are digested slowly and the amount of glucose available doesn't increase rapidly. This is not the case for foods containing a high amount of sugar, because far more insulin is produced to deal with the sudden rise and fall in blood glucose. A 'sugar rush' – where there is a sudden increase in blood glucose – can cause mood swings, hunger, headaches and tiredness, because a quantity of insulin is released to control the sudden rise in glucose. There is then too much insulin in the blood and not enough glucose, so we crave sweet foods that will rapidly raise our glucose levels again, which ultimately leads to weight gain.

Fibre

Fibre-rich foods, such as brown rice and wholewheat pasta, bran cereal and wholegrains, can help lower the risk of prediabetes, type 2 diabetes, stroke, cardiovascular disease, insulin resistance, obesity and **colorectal cancer**. Blood pressure and cholesterol levels can be significantly reduced by consuming a daily portion of oat bran, which also alleviates constipation. Foods high in dietary fibre are more filling, because the fibre absorbs fluid, providing bulk. This means that a fibre-rich meal will stay with you for longer, reducing hunger and helping with weight loss.

> **FACT: Diabetes UK states that adults in the UK only consume an average of 19g of fibre daily. The recommended daily amount of dietary fibre for those aged 16 years and upwards is 30g, but only 9% achieve this.**

> **FACT: Highly processed foods like white bread, bagels, muffins, crumpets and many processed breakfast cereals lack fibre, so they raise blood glucose quickly. Increasing your intake of fibre has a range of health benefits besides keeping blood glucose stable.**

Glycaemic index

Glycaemic index (GI) is a value assigned to carbohydrates based on how quickly or slowly they are digested to increase blood glucose levels. The glycaemic index was devised to rank foods that are digested quickly, causing a rapid increase in blood glucose over two hours, so that these foods can be avoided. Foods are rated out of 100, with white bread and pure sugar valued at 100, because they increase blood glucose so quickly. While a low GI diet will help to stabilise blood glucose levels, there is little evidence to show that this will help you lose weight.

Carbohydrates with a low glycaemic index score – usually 55 or less – are digested and absorbed more slowly, so blood glucose levels increase over a longer period. Chocolate, lactose (milk sugar) and fructose have low GI values, while sucrose (table sugar) has an intermediate to high GI value. Eating a diet that includes more low GI foods is associated with a reduced prediabetes and type 2 diabetes risk. Foods containing glucose are digested quickly and cause blood glucose and insulin levels to increase rapidly, so they have a high GI value greater than 70.

While only eating foods that don't cause a rapid increase in blood glucose based on GI values sounds like a great idea, trying to reduce diabetes risk using the GI value of foods can be complicated by various factors. For example:

- Blood glucose response is influenced by the combination of the GI value of different foods and the total amount of consumed carbohydrate.
- After eating unhealthy carbohydrates (such as white bread), high blood insulin levels then cause hunger and encourage fat storage.
- Eating low GI foods, such as cheese, together with carbohydrates (like bread), reduces the entire GI value of the sandwich, which is changed by the protein and fat in the cheese.
- The method of food preparation can change the GI value of certain foods. For example, whether it is fried in oil or grilled with no oil.

Carbohydrate-rich foods with the fibre content removed – white bread, white pasta and white rice – are highly processed and have the highest glycaemic index value, but various factors affect the glycaemic index of a food, so it can be difficult to rely on a low GI diet to keep blood glucose levels in the normal range.

BARBARA SAYS: *I have prediabetes and desperately want to lower the risk of it becoming type 2. I realised I was eating too much of the bad stuff – white bread, cake, biscuits, tinned fruit and ice cream. I know diabetes is all about controlling blood sugar because I have relatives with it, so I bought a glycaemic index guide. It's common sense, really. You know* *that a lemon is less sweet than a banana. It takes a bit of understanding, getting to grips with GI meal planning – basically not eating high sugar or white carb foods – but it's well worth understanding how what you eat can affect your glucose levels and I'm on the right track to a healthier lifestyle.*

FACT: The *British Medical Journal* has reported that eating five servings of dark (not milk) chocolate a week is linked to a 21% reduced risk of type 2 diabetes. Although dark chocolate – a low glycaemic index food – has a similar amount of energy and saturated fat as milk chocolate, high levels of flavonoids in dark chocolate offset the effects of saturated fat and sugar on weight gain, and the risk of prediabetes and type 2 diabetes.

Timing your meals

Whether your blood glucose levels are high or not, hormone levels tend to surge early in the morning – this is known as the **dawn phenomenon** – and blood glucose levels can also be harder to control the later it gets in the day, meaning it is never wise to eat a large meal late at night or before you go to bed. That means if you're trying to prevent or control prediabetes or type 2 diabetes, it does make a difference when you eat.

Controlling blood glucose with strict meal times involves having a larger breakfast, a moderate lunch and a lighter dinner at an earlier time – basically eating your meals within one 10-hour period in the day and not having anything out of this time-restricted period. For example, breakfast at 8.30 a.m., lunch at 1 p.m. dinner at 5.45 p.m. and finished by 6.30 p.m. Eating at regular times stabilises blood glucose levels, so consistency in the timing of your meals, in association with a healthy diet that is high in fibre, helps the body manage blood glucose effectively.

This method of controlling your blood glucose levels by following an eating plan is known as intermittent fasting. A 2014 study found that intermittent fasting improved prediabetes by reducing blood glucose levels by as much as 3–6% and increasing insulin efficiency by 20–31%, protecting against the onset of type 2 diabetes.

If you eat within a certain period of time, research has shown it can increase your metabolic rate by over 3.6%, reducing your appetite and calorie consumption, as well as improving your body's ability to burn calories and use food as fuel efficiently. However, having a specific timeframe for eating does not mean eating as much as you like within these parameters, because eating more calories than your body needs will cancel out the benefits of strict meal times. This method of weight loss and glucose control is a behaviour change that is easy to action, and has benefits such as reducing after-dinner snacking and making it easier to keep to a bedtime.

After as little as six weeks you should see noticeable improvements in insulin function and sensitivity, and appetite reduction and blood pressure. This suggests that sticking to regular timings for your meals may help with weight reduction and maintaining weight loss. This is especially helpful for people with prediabetes as it helps to restrict daily calories. Eating at specific times also has a positive effect on the hormones that help the breakdown of fat, meaning that more body fat is used for energy.

FACT: Raspberries are particularly good for people trying to avoid or reverse prediabetes. Research has shown that raspberries contain tannin and a substance that blocks the breakdown of starch, lowering blood glucose and blood insulin levels, as well as having a positive effect on cholesterol levels, insulin resistance and fasting plasma glucose levels. Eating 500ml of frozen raspberries reduces triglyceride blood fats after a high-carbohydrate, moderate fat meal (such as pasta with cheese sauce), making raspberries a useful tool in preventing prediabetes and type 2 diabetes if eaten regularly.

Stress

A certain amount of good stress is normal and necessary, but bad stress can have an adverse impact on your emotional and physical health. There is a link between stress-induced anxiety and depression, and an increase in blood glucose levels, and, although not a direct cause, there is evidence that stress can indirectly increase the risk of type 2 diabetes.

Stress is an inbuilt survival response, occurring as a reaction to a perceived threat that can be internal, in the form of your thoughts or emotions, or external. Increased blood flow is directed towards organs and muscles in preparation to protect you when faced with a threat, increasing your blood pressure and heart rate as your blood vessels constrict. Stored glucose is released by the liver to provide energy for 'the fight', but if you cannot respond to eliminate the issue, the stress continues and the glucose released to your muscles remains unused.

Stress is something that does not mix with diagnosed or undiagnosed prediabetes or type 2 diabetes as stress increases blood glucose, while emotional issues like depression and anxiety can prevent you from taking action to change your lifestyle (see chapter 8 for more on emotional health). All too often, stress provokes unhealthy behaviours like comfort eating, drinking more alcohol and smoking heavily. Stress also disrupts hormone levels, increasing blood pressure and reducing the action of insulin, which doesn't work well alongside the stress hormone, cortisol. Because insulin cannot work properly, blood glucose levels increase, making prediabetes and type 2 more likely to develop.

---

*❢ **ASHA SAYS:** I know it sounds obvious, but for much of my adult working life I've dealt with stress by comfort eating – a large bar of chocolate or takeaway in the evening to reward myself for getting through another stressful day. Now I'm paying the price. I didn't regard looking after my health as a priority and took it for granted until it was too late. For years I put my body under daily stress, meeting demanding work targets in the NHS – really prolonged stress. I would eat regular takeaways most nights as I was too tired and couldn't be bothered to cook, or I'd be working nights or be on call in a busy hospital and not be eating or sleeping regularly.*

I loved my job, but after almost 12 years of this I knew I'd been pushing my body too far with unhealthy food, not enough sleep and high stress levels. I was overweight and I was tested for prediabetes. The test came back positive and this was my wake-up call to make the necessary changes before I did any more damage to my body.

> **FACT: Cortisol encourages stored glucose to be released from the liver in the fight-or-flight response to stress.**

For people who are regularly stressed and do not deal with the emotion well, prediabetes and type 2 diabetes are a definite risk. Some react to stressful events and difficult periods in their life by drinking, eating and smoking more as a comforting coping mechanism. Stress is a common emotion, especially in the modern world. It is therefore important to remain healthy and reduce your chances of future ill-health triggered by stress in the following ways:

- Don't put too much pressure on yourself. Being a perfectionist adds to your ongoing stress levels.

- Pinpoint the source of your stress and think of ways this could be eased. If it's due to your job or family, identifying the problem is part of the solution to viewing the situation differently.

- Examine your reaction to the stress – do you easily fly off the handle or do you contain and try to control it so it eats away?

- Try to get enough sleep and exercise. Regular exercise helps reduce unhealthy cortisol levels, while a good period of sleep will reduce your stress levels.

- Try to avoid turning to eating, drinking or smoking more to help you get through a difficult time.

- Put some time aside for hobbies and leisure activities that relax you. This can divert your mind away from the stressful issue.

Medications and nutritional supplements

Some prescribed and over-the-counter products can prevent insulin from working correctly (if in doubt, consult your doctor), so you may be taking these medicines without realising that they are increasing your blood glucose levels:

- **Corticosteroid tablets**: Prescribed to manage inflammatory conditions, some corticosteroid tablets, and some corticosteroid creams used for skin conditions like eczema, will raise blood glucose levels.
- **Ginseng**: Although it encourages insulin production, ginseng also has a role in reducing cell longevity and cell death is one of the most common causes of loss of insulin-producing beta cells in the pancreas.
- **High blood pressure medications**: Atenolol, Bisoprolol, Minoxidil, Nifedipine and Amlodipine, all taken for high blood pressure, alter the way glucose is processed by the body.
- **Levothyroxine**: Used to treat an under-active thyroid gland (hypothyroidism), Levothyroxine increases blood glucose levels.
- **Octreotide**: Prescribed to help slow down the growth of cancer cells, this medication also slows down the production of hormones like insulin.
- **Oral diazoxide**: This drug is prescribed to prevent low blood glucose levels, so its purpose is to raise blood glucose levels. It works by inhibiting the pancreatic secretion of insulin.
- **Prednisone**: Used to prevent organ rejection after transplant, Prednisone destroys the insulin-producing cells of the pancreas so more insulin is required to control blood glucose levels.
- **Psychosis treatments**: Treatments such as Chlorpromazine, Promazine, Fluphenazine and Trifluoperazine are prescribed to manage mental disorder where thoughts and emotions are impaired, and they can increase blood glucose levels by affecting insulin production.
- **Statins**: Prescribed to people with high cholesterol levels, statins increase the risk of developing prediabetes and type 2 diabetes by raising blood glucose levels. If you have been prescribed statins you should continue to take them to reduce your risk of heart disease and stroke, but be aware of this potential side effect.

- **St John's Wort**: Mainly used as an over-the-counter remedy to treat mild or moderate depression, St John's Wort also impairs glucose tolerance by reducing insulin response. The unregulated use of this can be a risk factor for impaired glucose tolerance, insulin resistance and type 2 diabetes.
- **Thiazide**: This is a diuretic medicine prescribed to make you urinate more often, but increased urination decreases potassium levels in the body, resulting in higher blood glucose levels.
- **Vitamin B3**: Also known as nicotinic acid, vitamin B3 reduces insulin production, leading to higher blood glucose levels. It may be prescribed to treat high cholesterol levels or taken as an over-the-counter supplement containing B3 and other B vitamins.

If you have been prescribed any one of these medicines, it is obviously to treat and manage certain conditions. Never disregard professional medical advice or delay seeking it because of something you have read in this book and don't just stop taking your prescribed medicine, but if you are concerned about the increased risk of prediabetes or type 2 diabetes that taking any one of these medicines or supplements poses, speak to your doctor or other qualified health care professional.

The aim is to diagnose people at high risk of prediabetes as early as possible to prevent the progression to full-blown type 2. That progression depends on a number of factors, such as lifestyle changes and intervention with medications that effectively reduce blood glucose, such as metformin. Research has shown that for those with elevated glucose levels that are not high enough to be diagnosed as prediabetes, taking a prescribed glucose-lowering medicine like metformin returns glucose levels to within a normal range and reduces the risk of prediabetes developing.

BEVERLEY SAYS: *I was 12 stone, 5 pounds, and my doctor told me I was at high risk of type 2 diabetes due to my high blood glucose levels. At 60 years of age, the prospect of losing weight was not easy, but I managed over many months to get down to 11 stone. I was eating a low-calorie diet, but realised* *there was a lot of sugar in the diet foods and the yoghurts I bought, thinking they were healthy, so I stopped eating them and just ate normal meals in smaller portions. Although I've lost weight, my blood glucose levels continued to gradually increase. As a precaution, my doctor prescribed the diabetes medicine, metformin, and my glucose eventually levelled out to normal, but it took a while. I have to remain on the tablets, though, because my body either doesn't deal with glucose properly or I don't produce enough insulin as I get older, so I am effectively now a person living with type 2 diabetes.*

Medication to treat prediabetes is widely used in the US. Despite this, many questions remain about whether this is the most effective way to tackle this condition. For example, is it better to treat the outcome of an unhealthy lifestyle (high glucose levels and complications) with medication or tackle the root cause of elevated glucose levels with sustained lifestyle change?

One additional point is that while shorter-term than other factors that increase blood glucose levels, infections such as flu cause your body to release more glucose into the bloodstream as part of the body's defence mechanism to help fight the infection. This can happen even if you have no appetite or are eating less than usual. It is a completely normal reaction to an infection, but if you already have or are at risk from prediabetes or type 2 diabetes, it causes an additional, if temporary, increase in blood glucose levels.

Dehydration

The human body is 50% water, so when that percentage falls below 50% and the body is dehydrated it affects blood glucose levels. The amount of glucose doesn't actually increase due to lack of water, but the concentration of glucose in the blood increases, because the ratio of glucose to water has altered. Such blood glucose increases can range from mild to severe, but if you already have hyperglycaemia, this then becomes more pronounced.

Dehydration can occur for a number of reasons. Mild to moderate dehydration can result from intense exercise, hot weather and illness such as diarrhoea and vomiting. Severe dehydration reduces vital body electrolytes like sodium and potassium, which can be life-threatening. Symptoms that you are not getting enough water include headaches, feeling light-headed and dizzy, feeling tired with no energy, increased heart rate, low blood pressure, swelling in the hands and feet, muscle cramps, dark-coloured urine and having a dry mouth.

LINDA SAYS: *I was always busy at work, boosting my energy with sugary drinks. Although I knew these drinks weren't good for me, they were convenient, so I carried on for what must have been about two years. I noticed I often felt thirsty, although I just thought that was because everything was so hectic. One particularly busy day I had an awful headache and felt dizzy, which I put down to stress. I had a routine medical appointment and they measured my blood sugar, which led to a diagnosis of prediabetes. They also took a urine sample for testing, saying that my urine was very dark and concentrated, meaning my kidneys were working hard to remove the sugar from my body with very little water, so I was very dehydrated. I was also urinating quite a lot, so this made sense. A nurse told me that the symptoms were linked to the dehydration caused by the prediabetes. They told me I needed to take in more fluid. This news was scary and I knew I had to stop what I'd been doing. I started drinking water instead of sweet drinks for energy, making sure I did this throughout the day. After several weeks of doing things differently I stopped feeling thirsty and urinating a lot. I went back to the nurse for a check-up and she told me that by managing the prediabetes I had stopped the dehydration and allowed my body to bring sugar levels down to normal.*

It may be difficult to calculate how much water you actually need to drink, but six to eight glasses spread over one day is a good rule of thumb. Drinking water when you are thirsty is adequate for most people to replenish what is lost. Avoid drinks or juices loaded with sugar or glucose, like non-diet drinks, energy drinks and fruit juices. If you're already dehydrated, caffeine-based drinks like coffee, tea and diet cola are a bad idea, because they make you urinate more frequently.

Caffeine

Blood glucose levels are affected by caffeine in tea, coffee, cola drinks, chocolate and energy drinks. For people without elevated blood glucose levels, caffeine provides a pick-me-up, but if you have undiagnosed or diagnosed prediabetes or type 2 diabetes it can increase glucose levels. This is because caffeine lowers insulin sensitivity and people with insulin resistance react to caffeine in a different way to those without the condition.

For those who already have prediabetes or type 2 diabetes, caffeine can raise both glucose and insulin levels, where more insulin is released in response to high glucose levels. Researchers found that when people with type 2 diabetes took a 250mg caffeine pill at breakfast and another at lunchtime (the equivalent of drinking two cups of coffee with each meal), their blood glucose level was 8% higher than on days when they didn't have caffeine. Their glucose level also increased by more after each meal, because caffeine affects how the body responds to insulin.

It is thought that caffeine has this effect, because it increases stress hormones such as epinephrine (also known as adrenaline) and cortisol, which can prevent body cells from using too much glucose and may also prevent more insulin from being produced. Caffeine changes the action of a chemical called **adenosine**, which has a controlling effect on the amount of insulin produced by the body and how body cells respond to it. Because caffeine is a stimulant, it also has an impact on sleep and a lack of sleep has a negative effect on insulin sensitivity or how well the body's cells are able to use insulin.

Blood glucose levels are affected by as little as two cups of percolated coffee or four cups of black tea per day – that's around 200 milligrams of caffeine. However, the reaction to caffeine is individual, depending on factors such as age and weight, so some may have no problems with increased glucose levels and this amount of caffeine, while others react to far less than 200 milligrams. If you are a regular coffee drinker it is also possible to build up tolerance to caffeine over time, so blood glucose levels won't necessarily rise if you have prediabetes or type 2 diabetes and drink a couple of cups of tea or coffee each day.

A Harvard study suggesting that caffeine can actually lower blood glucose levels found that having one more cup of coffee than is usually consumed each day may reduce the risk of developing type 2 diabetes by 37%. However, those who drank one cup of coffee less per day increased their type 2 risk by 17% and it was the same for those drinking tea. Surprisingly, the same study showed that decaffeinated coffee also increased blood glucose levels in the same way as caffeinated coffee.

Pain

When chronic pain, such as back pain or arthritis, is present that cannot be managed with pain relief, this often leads to elevated blood glucose levels. Experiencing pain can also raise levels of stress hormones, which in turn increases insulin resistance and elevates blood glucose levels. The inflammation associated with conditions such as chronic arthritis or injury causes greater insulin resistance and insulin resistance in turn leads to inflammation. Due to inflammation, blood glucose levels can rise higher and higher, eventually resulting in type 2 diabetes. Emotional stress can also increase levels of the chemicals associated with inflammation.

When pain is present a stress response triggers hormones to be released that mobilise stored energy. These, in turn, lead to chronic high glucose levels. Research has shown that acute severe pain reduces insulin sensitivity by affecting the processes that use or store glucose. Painful trauma triggers disturbances in these processes and the body's ability to react to insulin, increasing blood glucose levels. If you have constant or frequent severe pain due to a medical condition such as arthritis, you could also be living with increased blood glucose levels due to a combination of pain and pain medication.

There is a significant association between prediabetes and chronic pain symptoms. It is now recognised that prediabetes, obesity, insulin resistance and metabolic syndrome are risk factors for peripheral neuropathy (severe nerve pain) in the hands, feet and legs, and peripheral neuropathy is a major contributor to reduced quality of life due to pain. Persistent high blood glucose levels damage the nerves over time. Studies have shown that people with prediabetes are also at increased risk of **sensory polyneuropathy** – decreased ability to move and feel due to damage to multiple nerves – before the onset of full-blown type 2.

If you already have nerve pain in either your feet, legs or hands, lifestyle changes to increase the amount of exercise you do can help to manage neuropathy pain by reducing blood glucose levels. There is no available medication to reverse nerve damage, but exercise-based lifestyle change has shown promising results in enhancing peripheral nerve regeneration in the hands and feet.

- Whether you have a diagnosis of prediabetes or type 2 diabetes or not, begin a regular exercise routine to actively reduce your blood glucose and nerve pain.
- Keep a behaviour change diary of your progress with regular exercise to reduce your blood glucose levels and nerve pain. If you have a blood glucose meter, record your results to track your changes – you will see a definite reduction in glucose levels and also nerve pain.

WHAT IS A BLOOD GLUCOSE METER?

A blood glucose meter is a device that helps you manage diabetes by measuring your blood glucose levels via a finger prick test. The need for a meter depends on your specific medical condition and treatment. It is essential for people whose diabetes is being treated with insulin, but not everyone needs to monitor their blood glucose levels regularly. If you want to know if a meter could help your specific circumstances, ask your healthcare professional.

As I think you will now appreciate, there is a wide range of factors that can affect blood glucose levels, but I hope you now have a better understanding of what can raise and – generally more importantly – lower them.

Lowering blood pressure and blood cholesterol

Diabetes and high blood pressure are closely linked, frequently co-occurring and often worsening the effects of one another. High blood pressure (hypertension) is more common in people with diabetes and it can exacerbate the damage diabetes causes to blood vessels and the heart. Reducing raised blood pressure is another key change to effectively lower your risk of prediabetes and type 2 diabetes.

- Currently, how do you think your blood pressure impacts your overall health?
- Do you know what your blood cholesterol level is?
- What could you do to make a difference to these readings?

People who already have prediabetes or type 2 diabetes are advised to reduce their blood pressure to prevent damage to the heart, and the body's small (*microvascular*) and large (*macrovascular*) blood vessels. Reducing your blood pressure also appears to have a preventative role in type 2 diabetes – high blood pressure (hypertension) being one of the group of metabolic syndrome factors or health problems that put you at risk of type 2 diabetes (*see* chapter 3).

> **FACT: Lowering systolic blood pressure by 5 mmHg has been shown to reduce the risk of developing type 2 diabetes by 16%.**

Losing weight, taking regular exercise and removing excess salt from your diet will reduce your blood pressure. Being overweight or obese is a significant risk factor for high blood pressure. Excess weight, especially around the abdomen, can strain the heart and blood vessels, leading to increased blood pressure. Your doctor may also prescribe medication to reduce your blood pressure.

High blood pressure medication (anti-hypertensives) such as angiotensin-converting enzyme (ACE) inhibitors and angiotensin II receptor blockers (ARBs) are already prescribed to millions of people to reduce the risk of heart disease and stroke. These same medications can also reduce the risk of developing insulin resistance and type 2 diabetes. As we have seen, lowering systolic blood pressure by 5mmHg – achievable with medication and lifestyle changes – can reduce the risk of type 2 diabetes by as much as 16%.

> **RIZWANA SAYS:** *I had a heart attack in 2021 that was partly caused by high blood pressure. That is when I first became aware that I had heart disease, despite knowing about a number of risk factors, like prediabetes, obesity and my ethnicity. My consultant told me that 70% of people who have heart attacks also have high blood pressure. I have now made changes to my lifestyle, such as taking regular exercise, eating a healthy diet and reducing my stress levels with yoga. My heart health is now very good, my blood pressure and blood glucose are in the normal range, and my prediabetes has been reversed, so it should not progress to type 2 diabetes.*

Having both diabetes and high blood pressure strongly increases the chance of developing other serious health conditions, such as heart attack and stroke. Even before prediabetes is diagnosed elevated blood glucose levels over time will have a negative effect on the body. Excess glucose is filtered from the blood into the urine as a waste product, causing damage and scarring to kidney tissues. This damage interferes with your kidney filtration function, leading to salt and water retention, which raises blood pressure. Continually elevated blood glucose levels damage small blood vessels, affecting their function. This also contributes to high blood pressure. It is therefore important to speak to your doctor about how to reduce and manage high blood pressure.

Reducing your cholesterol level is also a key change you can make for better health, and with the right advice and support you can reduce harmful blood fats. Scientists have now discovered that the levels of 184 different fat molecules in the blood can help to predict those individuals at highest risk of developing prediabetes, type 2 diabetes and cardiovascular disease, years before symptoms appear, so these conditions can be prevented through lifestyle change measures.

High cholesterol levels (blood fats) have also been linked to high blood pressure and type 2 diabetes. Studies show that increased cholesterol levels can lead to insulin resistance, and they have a role in triggering prediabetes and metabolic syndrome. Cholesterol travels in the blood in two different ways:

- LDL cholesterol (low-density lipoprotein) is known as 'bad cholesterol', because it forms the majority of blood fats in the body, and elevated LDL cholesterol levels increase the risk of heart disease and stroke.
- HDL cholesterol (high-density lipoprotein) is known as 'good cholesterol', because it removes other forms of harmful fats from the blood and carries them back to the liver.

There is also another type of fat in the blood known as **triglycerides**, which the body uses for energy. Although triglycerides and HDL cholesterol are beneficial to the body, the combination of high levels of triglycerides and/or good and bad cholesterol can increase the risk of stroke and heart attack due to having high overall blood fats.

> **FACT: High levels of HDL cholesterol can lower your risk of heart disease and stroke.**

Research has found that consuming too much dietary sugar can lower levels of HDL (good) cholesterol and raise the amount of LDL (bad) cholesterol and triglycerides. When there is too much LDL cholesterol in the body it can build up on the walls of blood vessels and is known as plaque (not to be confused with the plaque that forms on teeth, a sticky substance that contains bacteria formed from food particles and saliva). Narrowing caused by plaque forming on the artery walls reduces blood flow, eventually leading to heart disease and stroke.

SURESH SAYS: *It's so easy to let your cholesterol levels creep up when you have prediabetes, or just to think of it as something you should keep an eye on. I had no idea cholesterol wasn't just connected to poor diet and little exercise. My doctor explained that smoking and alcohol affect cholesterol levels, too. I was smoking too much and drinking most days in the evenings to relax with the stress of my job, but now I realise that you can't do that long term: my health is far more* *important. Now I've cut right back on alcohol and cigarettes, and aim to stop smoking completely. My last cholesterol test showed this was having a positive effect. My total cholesterol has come down from 8.4 to 5.5, which is a real improvement, and my blood glucose levels have also come down.*

It is possible to lower the risk of high cholesterol with certain actions, such as reducing the amount of saturated fat that you eat by making healthier food choices and by quitting smoking. Smoking can raise your cholesterol level and also increases the risk of having serious health problems like heart disease, stroke and cancer. For people who already have high triglyceride and LDL cholesterol levels, there are medications that can bring this under control, so speak to your doctor if you are concerned about this. The good news is, there are positive actions you can take to address high cholesterol levels:

- Choose foods that are low in saturated fats and trans-fats – these are found in commercial baked goods like biscuits, cakes and pies, and fried foods, such as French fries, doughnuts and fried chicken.
- Choose lean meats, fat-free or low-fat milk, yoghurt and cheese, wholegrains, fruits and vegetables.
- Choose foods that do not contain added sugar and are low in sodium (salt). Avoid adding salt to cooking and to meals.
- Choose foods that are high in fibre. This helps reduce cholesterol levels and does not cause a sharp rise in blood glucose.

TIP

Always read food labels as foods that are high in saturated fats also tend to be high in cholesterol. Check the red, yellow and green traffic light system on the front of the packaging, which shows fat and sugar content, but look at the ingredients label on the back, too. If ingredients such as palm oil, sugar, glucose or sodium are listed within the first three ingredients, avoid that food.

When there is persistent high blood glucose over time, the liver is forced to store any excess glucose as visceral fat around body organs, such as the liver and kidneys, raising cholesterol levels and increasing the risk of developing insulin resistance. Here are some things you can do to help:

- Write down the steps you take in your behaviour change diary and chart your progress.

- Have your blood fats measured regularly. This can be done in some larger pharmacies rather than by having to book an appointment at your doctor's surgery.

- Focus on a heart-healthy lifestyle by eating more fruit, vegetables and wholegrains, and try yoga to lower your stress levels to reduce blood pressure and blood cholesterol levels.

- Change your diet and increase the amount of exercise you do as this impacts on blood pressure and blood cholesterol.

- Set yourself small, achievable goals, such as reducing your blood pressure by 5mm/Hg – a proven way to significantly reduce your risk of prediabetes and type 2 diabetes.

Stopping smoking

Smoking and diabetes don't mix, significantly increasing the chances of heart and blood vessel disease. See your doctor as soon as possible for help and support with quitting a nicotine addiction. Everyone is aware that smoking is associated with health problems, but it is especially harmful when you have insulin resistance. Smoking raises cholesterol levels and can double the risk of having a stroke and circulatory problems. It can also double the chances of developing the kidney disease (nephropathy) and erectile dysfunction associated with high blood glucose levels.

- Do you smoke as a coping mechanism because it calms you when life gets stressful or because you enjoy it? Think about why you smoke and whether those reasons have changed since you started smoking.

- Have you tried to quit smoking before? What caused you to begin again?

- Have you tried, or considered, getting help from your doctor to stop smoking?

> **JUDITH SAYS:** *I smoked from the age of 16 and I think this was because all my friends were doing it. In my 30s, I began to experience health issues, like a hacking cough and being short of breath, as well as being diagnosed with prediabetes. I then had an accident at work and had to rest, so I wasn't even moving about much. I was on half pay and the cost of my habit was something I began to really notice. After a few months, I just had to admit to myself that to carry on smoking was too expensive. I sought help to quit from the NHS Quit Smoking app to manage my cravings and track my progress. If I'm truthful, my motivation was initially to save money, but then, as I saw the health benefits, it became stopping smoking to be healthier. I now haven't smoked for 15 months. I have a better quality of life and I don't have prediabetes any more either.*

The sooner you stop smoking, the sooner your body can begin to repair the damage smoking has done to your cells. Insulin becomes more effective at lowering blood glucose levels after only eight weeks of not smoking. Quitting smoking is an important prevention change you can make, as smoking has now been identified as an independent risk factor for type 2 diabetes and, for people with prediabetes, the risk of developing chronic complications like heart and nerve disease is made worse by smoking.

Once you stop smoking your body will begin to repair itself almost immediately. You will notice the following benefits to your health:

- After 20 minutes without smoking your pulse rate returns to normal.
- After eight hours your oxygen levels improve and your blood carbon monoxide level reduces by half.
- By 48 hours all traces of carbon monoxide are gone and your lungs clear themselves of mucus, so your sense of smell and taste becomes much sharper.

- After 72 hours you have more energy and the bronchial passages to your lungs start to relax, making breathing feel much easier.
- From two to 12 weeks after giving up smoking your heart and muscles start receiving blood much more efficiently due to improved blood circulation.
- After three to nine months your lung capacity will have increased by 10% and any breathlessness, wheezing or cough will be easing.
- After one year without cigarettes your risk of having a heart attack will now be halved compared with someone who still smokes.
- After 10 years your risk of death from lung cancer will now be halved compared with someone who still smokes.

FACT: Research shows that risk of type 2 diabetes is increased in people who smoke and the higher the number of daily cigarettes, the greater the risk. Cigarette smokers are 30–40% more likely to develop type 2 diabetes than non-smokers.

If you are considering quitting a nicotine habit, this is to be applauded – it takes a lot of courage to admit that you want to quit. This will significantly reduce your risk of developing prediabetes and type 2 diabetes, and majorly benefit your health. You will feel much better, be able to breathe easier and have more energy. Quitting is a process and you are bound to have some setbacks, but as part of your lifestyle change, plan smoke-free activities with others, like going for walks or trying new hobbies. It might take time, but you will get there in the end!

As we have seen, smoking is not an option if you have insulin resistance – meaning raised blood glucose levels, prediabetes, type 2 diabetes, metabolic syndrome or any other form of diabetes. Nicotine vapes (e-cigarettes) can help you to significantly reduce or stop smoking cigarettes, and they are substantially less harmful, although vaping can still cause insulin resistance. Vaping is recommended by the NHS for adult smokers who wish to quit, but vaping is not a harmless activity as e-cigarettes still contain nicotine and caffeine, substances that raise glucose levels. Few studies have been carried out to examine the health outcomes of vaping. The healthiest option is clearly not to smoke or vape at all, so, if you are vaping to quit smoking, you should aim to eventually stop vaping, too.

No one expects you to give up nicotine with just sheer willpower and no practical help or encouragement. Talk to your doctor for advice and support or call a telephone quit line for real-time expert help. There are also online resources available to support you as you try to quit cigarettes for good. Nicotine replacement products such as gum, patches and lozenges are some of the best tools to help you stop smoking. These proven ways to quit can double your chances of stopping for good.

Going to medical appointments

If you sometimes miss the opportunity to attend a routine medical appointment, making sure you attend future appointments is another key change you can make. Although sometimes appointments can seem to be a waste of your time, health professionals (including dentists and opticians when you have a check-up) do record your health status since you were last seen, so these results are in the system.

Prediabetes is often first recognised as a risk to health at a routine medical appointment. As we have already seen, not everyone with prediabetes will go on to develop type 2 diabetes, although if blood glucose levels have been increased for some time there is a high risk of complications developing, such as eye, kidney, nerve and heart problems.

- Do you sometimes cancel a medical appointment because you are just too busy to attend?

- Or is the reason you don't go because the travel is too costly, you are fearful of the outcome or it's simply too much effort?

- Do you sometimes feel that you don't get much out of some appointments, because you see a different health professional each time and have to spend time explaining your medical history?

For people who have already been diagnosed with prediabetes or type 2 diabetes, attending regular health appointments helps you to lose more weight and reduce blood glucose levels. Shared medical appointments with others who also have the condition are now available for people with prediabetes to provide ongoing group support, nutritional advice and care.

❝ DEAN SAYS: *I'm 58 and run a newspaper distribution business, so early mornings are very stressful and I'm on my feet all day. I was overweight and felt unfit, and I was getting pins and needles in my lower legs, but I put that down to long hours standing up. I also noticed that I needed to visit the bathroom several times a night, disturbing my wife Lisa as well. I constantly felt tired, so I stopped having a cup of tea in the evenings and tried to get to bed earlier. I was concerned about my health, but I pushed it to the back of my mind.*

This went on for almost two years, but one day I got out of bed, and my left foot felt numb and cold. I went to work as normal, but finally found time to make a doctor's appointment. I was apprehensive about what my doctor might say. In fact, I almost cancelled my appointment, telling myself that the feeling in my foot would come back, but I knew it was just fear, so I made myself go.

When I saw the doctor I was really relieved that he listened and didn't judge me for not coming sooner. Instead, he examined my foot and did some tests, including a HbA1c test. I had another blood test after fasting all night and going without breakfast, and both tests showed a high level of glucose in my blood (12.9mmol/L and 13.6mml/L instead of the usual normal level of 6mmol/L (or below). My doctor diagnosed type 2 diabetes, but said it could be treated with diet and exercise.

I wasn't really shocked by the diagnosis. I was just relieved that I now had an answer. Lisa was very supportive, and we planned how we could eat a better diet and make the time for walks during the week. The planning was the easy part, but

> *putting the plan into action took more effort because we both work irregular hours, but we knew it was the way to improve my health.*
>
> *When I had my type 2 diabetes appointment a few weeks later, I was able to report the changes I had made to my routine and lifestyle. I had a finger prick blood glucose test, which showed a reading of 7.5mmol/L. This was a snapshot in time, rather than an HbA1c test showing blood glucose levels over three months, but it was a huge improvement. I was advised to keep up the good work and told to attend the clinic every six months to monitor my progress. I was also sleeping better, only needed to get up occasionally to use the bathroom and the numbness in my foot had vastly improved.*
>
> *I wasn't at all anxious about my next diabetes clinic appointment. I knew I had been looking after myself, because my foot felt normal again with no numbness, and I no longer needed to get up in the night. I felt well for the first time in ages, and both me and Lisa had lost around 14 pounds.*

Many people only see a doctor if they feel unwell, so they may go years between appointments. If you are generally healthy you may not be invited to attend routine health checks where symptoms of prediabetes or type 2 diabetes could be spotted. It is often the case that the effects of raised blood glucose levels are first detected during appointments with the dentist, dental hygienist or optician rather than a doctor, as these health professionals tend to be visited more regularly.

As we have already seen, gum disease and tooth decay are more common in people with prediabetes and type 2 diabetes as a consequence of higher blood glucose levels. Bacteria in the mouth are attracted to the glucose, causing damage to teeth and gums. This is also the case for people who do not yet know they have prediabetes or type 2 diabetes, so a visit to the dentist is an excellent opportunity to prevent diabetes. Just a reminder: according to Diabetes UK, as many as

850,000 people currently live with undiagnosed prediabetes and type 2, while a further 13.6 million people are at risk from these conditions.

> **ANIKA SAYS:** *I went to my dentist for a check-up and he commented that my gumline looked a bit sore. I told him it had been like that for three months, but I only noticed the soreness when I brushed my teeth. He suggested that I see my doctor, feeling the cause might need to be investigated. I did just that and had a blood test that revealed high sugar levels. It was really quite surprising as I don't have type 2 diabetes in my family and I didn't think I was at risk of getting it. I'm now changing what I eat to cut down on sugar – especially avoiding fruit juices and smoothies – to help my teeth and my weight, and trying to be more active. I've got a follow-up blood test soon, so hopefully that will reflect the changes I've made.*

Opticians already refer people with hyperglycaemia-related eye issues to their doctor for further investigation, while dentists can also utilise any medical treatment records to help diagnose and access support for people to manage prediabetes. Hopefully, the involvement of opticians and dentists will enable more people to be diagnosed with prediabetes at an earlier stage, before type 2 diabetes becomes established, helping to reduce serious long-term complications of high blood glucose levels.

If you have to cancel a medical appointment, you will be sent another one, so there is no getting away from them! Try to see attending these appointments as something you can do to help yourself, to ensure you remain as healthy as possible. This is especially the case if you have prediabetes or type 2 diabetes.

Make changes permanent

I can only be honest here and tell you that taking action to change your behaviour and your lifestyle won't be easy, but it's definitely worth taking on the challenge and making the effort, because you really can reduce your risk, prevent or reverse prediabetes and type 2 diabetes. Success is well within your grasp, just remember:

- **Start small**: Begin with manageable changes and gradually build on them.

- **Monitor progress**: Track how well you're doing to stay motivated and identify areas that might need improvement.

- **Be patient**: Change takes time and setbacks are to be expected.

- **Get support**: Ask your family, friends and health professionals for support, encouragement and guidance.

- **Think long term**: Avoid quick-fix diets or health kicks and focus on sustainable lifestyle changes.

✶ Key messages ✶

- Lifestyle change to incorporate healthy eating, physical activity and a modest reduction in body weight into your life can prevent and delay prediabetes and type 2 diabetes for those at risk of these conditions.

- Increased physical activity is especially beneficial for weight reduction: two and a half hours of brisk walking at a moderate intensity per week reduces diabetes risk by 27%, independent of your body weight. Regular exercise reduces the risk of developing type 2 diabetes by up to 40%.

- Weight-loss drugs are not a magic bullet to solve obesity. This can only be done successfully with lifestyle changes to improve long-term health. You may not need to lose weight, but you may still be at risk of prediabetes and type 2 diabetes. One of the benefits of being more active is that it will help you reduce this risk.

- Reducing systolic blood pressure by 5 mmHg has been shown to reduce the risk of developing type 2 diabetes by 16%.

- Cigarette smokers are 30–40% more likely to develop type 2 diabetes than non-smokers.

Chapter 8

Emotional health

This chapter acknowledges the emotional impact of a diabetes diagnosis and, with a particular emphasis on positive mental health, provides advice on how to self-manage your diabetes in the long term.

So far this book has largely focused on the physical aspects of having prediabetes and type 2 diabetes, but I want to close by looking at the psychological aspects of diabetes, because it is vital to consider those, too. Why are the psychological aspects important? Well, because your emotional health, such as how well you feel you can cope with diabetes, directly affects your ability to manage the condition. This should never be ignored or underestimated, because poor emotional health has physical consequences. Sustained stress can lead to inflammatory changes throughout the body, and can also worsen heart disease and depression. In fact, inflammation is especially common in those with long-term elevated glucose levels, and not only has a negative effect on prediabetes and type 2 diabetes, but also worsens arthritis, osteoporosis, some cancers, and tooth and gum disease. Negative emotions also impact the immune response, prolonging infections such as flu, delaying wound healing, especially when blood circulation is impaired, and, again, raising blood glucose levels.

Responding to a diagnosis

Disbelief, distress, resentment, fear, anger, self-blame – a diagnosis of prediabetes, type 2 diabetes or complications may bring with it many negative emotions. If you've been feeling over-tired or needing to urinate more frequently the diagnosis might come as a relief, because at least now you have an explanation for those symptoms, but, particularly if you have had no symptoms and the condition has been discovered by chance, it can be extremely upsetting.

> **RITA SAYS:** *It was a complete shock to be told I had type 2 diabetes, especially when it was explained what that would mean for the rest of my life. I didn't take it all in for months. I felt ashamed, judged and labelled. Fortunately, my sister is a counsellor and I talked it out with her. She helped me see that these feelings are totally normal and that I shouldn't blame myself or my body. I've now changed my mindset about diabetes. It's not "poor me" any more, it's now a feeling of gratitude that I have this diagnosis, and can do something to manage it and perhaps even reverse it.*

Similar to the bereavement response, you may go through different stages – anger, apathy, denial, bargaining – before you come to terms with and accept that you have a complex health condition. This realisation marks the beginning of a new way of living for you. As discussed previously, you will need to adopt a new mindset and make some changes to the way you live your life (see chapters 6 and 7), but in terms of your emotional health you may find this challenging – most people do.

❝**JESS SAYS:** *It was so overwhelming when I was first diagnosed with type 2 diabetes. I had to come to terms with the news, try to make changes to my lifestyle, remember to take medicines at the right time and in the right amount, and learn about carbohydrates and the effects of exercise. It went on and on. I slowly began to incorporate changes into my life, but still felt as though I wasn't doing enough and that my doctor might tell me off. I read as much as I could about managing diabetes and how to go about it. My family gave me support, too, and everyone joined in, so we ate healthier meals and all tried to do some regular exercise. This made things a lot easier, so I felt like I could manage it all. Now, six months on, I think we are all healthier for me having diabetes and my doctor is very pleased with the results.*❞

I realise it is impossible to accept having diabetes with open arms, but being positive about your health releases feel-good hormones and stops you being stressed. Your brain produces thoughts and emotions conducive to dealing with situations in a practical way, making you relaxed and optimistic about overcoming any challenge. This is conveyed to your body as positive energy, because the information you have received is transmitted to every single nerve cell in your body. Remember that thoughts and emotions are made of energy, and if you have negative feelings about any aspect of your diabetes, or any issue generally, this bad energy is physically reflected in the form of poor health.

❝**KATHIE'S STORY:** *For the first few months after my prediabetes diagnosis I was really anxious that I might be making the condition worse, so that it turned into type 2 diabetes, and I felt stressed, because I was always busy, but had to remember lots of health things, too. However, I eventually realised that feeling I was hard done by and missing out was a negative way* *of thinking, so I decided to think positively about the situation. I had this condition and it was part of my life now. I realised that I felt OK with that and it didn't really bother me that I had to make a few changes to accommodate prediabetes.*

I wasn't prescribed any diabetes medication, just advised to eat well and exercise more, but I can honestly say that being positive and not seeing having prediabetes as an enemy made a huge difference. When I had my first HbA1c blood test to diagnose prediabetes the result was 8.5mmol/L. By eating a healthier diet with fewer unhealthy snacks, and walking to and from work (about two miles a day), plus a positive attitude about my overall health, physical and emotional, my next HbA1c reading six months later was 5mmol/L. I had achieved a normal blood glucose reading from making a few very minor changes.

Making ongoing lifestyle changes for prediabetes and type 2 diabetes can certainly negatively impact mood, leading to stress, anxiety and depression. This can then become a cycle where poor emotional health can worsen diabetes management. Continual demands, such as diet, exercise and taking medicine at the right times, can be burdensome, while poor diabetes control causes sharp glucose fluctuations that directly affect mood, causing irritability or depression.

The strategies that will help your emotional health are very similar to those that support your physical health, but setbacks, as we have seen in Part I, are common when making any change to your lifestyle, but it is important to learn from them and keep moving forward. Don't blame or criticise yourself, look at why you were blown off course and reset your health goals, perhaps breaking them down into more manageable and achievable aims. Seek encouragement and guidance from health professionals, friends and family, too.

The brain is continually influenced by chemical processes and fluctuating blood glucose levels impact your thoughts, decisions and subsequent diabetes self-management behaviours. This is due to changes in the brain that occur with high glucose levels, leading to a reduced ability to cope with difficulties, such as the pressures of work, or the ups and downs of the daily routine, leading to the perception that these events are more stressful. In 2018, Public Health England did some research that quantified the psychological impact of elevated glucose levels. This showed that:

- Three in five people (64%) living with diabetes said they had experienced psychological or emotional health problems as a result of their condition.

- Only three in 10 people living with diabetes agreed they definitely felt in control of their condition.

- One in five people living with diabetes had sought support or counselling from a trained professional to help them manage their diabetes.

SUZANNE SAYS: *Being diagnosed with diabetes is like suddenly having a new child to care for and that child is constantly demanding your attention. Type 2 diabetes seemed to have taken over my life, but I'm slowly coming to terms with it and learning how to adapt, so I can keep as healthy as possible for as long as possible. The changes I am making to my meals and exercise routine are changes I've needed to make for a very long time, and I have accepted this as positive and good. You just have to give yourself some time to adapt.*

One of the reasons a prediabetes or diabetes diagnosis can have such an impact on your emotional health is because, as someone with diabetes, you largely have to manage the condition yourself. Your doctor may check up on you periodically or you may have regular appointments with the diabetes nurse at your doctor's practice. Helplines and support groups are also available, but whether you have been prescribed medication or not, you will undertake around 95% of your diabetes care yourself. This inevitably places a lot of stress on the individual. Of course, some people are better able to cope with diabetes self-care than others, but you should never feel that you can't ask for help and you can always talk to your doctor or other health professionals about your diabetes and any emotional concerns.

❦ HASSAN SAYS: A few years ago I was diagnosed with type 2 diabetes. I'd been feeling tired and depressed for ages, in a rut and not wanting to do anything. Over several years I'd put on lots of weight and was really unfit. I weighed 18 stone at the age of 37 – and I'm a short bloke. My main "hobby" was drinking and smoking in front of the TV. As well as depression, I had anxiety, panic attacks, heart palpitations and high cholesterol.

My doctor arranged a blood test which showed high sugar and I was put on medicine for that, too. My liver wasn't working well because of the drinking and this made me feel worse. I can't say that there was anything that made me want to change, other than feeling terrible all the time. I just suddenly decided it was time to do things differently. I owed it to myself.

I stopped eating high-carbohydrate food, and stopped drinking and smoking. I kept a record of what I was doing on my computer so I could see my progress and this really motivated me to keep going. I recorded my weight each time I was weighed at the hospital and my blood results. I didn't write down what I ate or the exercise I took, but gave myself a pat on the back when I ate in a healthy way and exercised. I only recorded the times I found my routine hard to stick to and why. I know it isn't wise to do it all at once, but once I'd decided what I had to do I was suddenly so determined that I wanted to make changes that mattered. I set myself a timeframe of two months, up until my next diabetes review, when I was shocked to find that my sugar levels had halved from making these changes. The doctor was very pleased and congratulated me for taking things in hand.

My weight was down to 15 stone 7 pounds, and the doctor took me off the glucose-lowering and cholesterol medicine. I was also feeling so much brighter, with no symptoms of depression, and my anxiety had gone, too, because my success improved my mood. My blood glucose and cholesterol tests were within the normal range, and blood tests showed that my liver was working well. I was so pleased that all my efforts had paid off and I was feeling healthy again. This spurred me on to lose more weight and to continue the good work.

I did have cravings for cigarettes and alcohol, but instead I took a walk or used my treadmill. It wasn't always easy, but I didn't want to go back to my old ways. I walked every day and began to eat some more healthy carbohydrates, like porridge, or jacket potato with chilli – foods to provide energy, but not increase my glucose levels too rapidly. I now weigh 12 stone 10 pounds and I feel really well, with no signs of depression or anxiety. It seems as though getting diagnosed with type 2 diabetes was a blessing in disguise and I can truly say I've never felt this healthy and fit.

DIABETES BURNOUT

There is a state of mind known as 'diabetes burnout', which describes feeling frustrated and overwhelmed by having to manage your diabetes. Diabetes burnout can lead people to ignore their diabetes for a while until they feel ready to cope with it again. These burnouts can be minor or major and they last for a few hours, a few days or even a few months.

Health professionals now recognise that, psychologically speaking, it is normal for people with diabetes or prediabetes to struggle with their condition and that some may consider not looking after their diabetes to keep glucose levels under control. While this is a perfectly understandable way of thinking, diabetes tends to need even more attention if it is ignored for too long and the truth is that if you don't look after your diabetes it will almost certainly come back and bite you.

Overcoming diabetes burnout is about recognising why you feel fed up and acknowledging that your feelings about having prediabetes or diabetes are based on emotions rather than permanent situations. Emotions can change very quickly, so you may feel fed up one day, but able to cope and manage the next. However, if the feeling that you can't cope with your prediabetes, diabetes or complications persists, it is important to talk to a health professional to work out how you can move past a stage of finding things hard to a state where you feel in control.

Managing diabetes

Research shows that due to the stress of managing the condition yourself and the increasing number of diabetes-related health issues you will probably encounter, the impact of diabetes on emotional health tends to rise the longer you've had the condition. That being so, I hope you understand that however long you've had prediabetes or type 2 diabetes it's normal to feel stressed, depressed or overwhelmed by it. The impact of high blood glucose levels on mood also contributes to these feelings, but rest assured that there are several strategies which will make a difference.

First of all, don't let your life revolve around your diabetes. It is very easy to find that much of your attention and many of your thoughts are directed towards managing your prediabetes or diabetes, but don't let that happen – make sure you also live your life as well as you possibly can. Having said that, it makes sense to learn as much as you can about diabetes. Reading this book is a positive start to informing yourself about the condition, but even if you've had prediabetes or type 2 diabetes for years, there is always new information to discover. Keeping up with new thinking and scientific developments can feel like a chore, but it's worth doing, because it puts you in control.

If you do experience burnout, to whatever degree, work out why it has happened. What has caused you to want to give up on self-care? There can be many reasons, including life pressures, the responsibility, routine, boredom, depression and so on. Recognising the underlying reason can help to address the problem. Don't give up everything you enjoy – if you feel like you're missing out, it won't help and will only make you miserable – and above all, be kind to yourself and recognise that you will have good days and bad days. There is no one with fantastically well-controlled diabetes all the time, so don't feel that your self-management efforts aren't good enough if your test results aren't 'perfect'. If you had perfect blood results every time they were tested, you wouldn't have diabetes!

Mindfulness

It is possible to improve your emotional health over time using focused mindfulness to change your negative thought patterns. This method draws on **neuroplasticity**, the ability of the brain, in response to your thoughts, to form new networks and different connections. This reprogramming results in changes in how the brain tells us what to do. Throughout your life, neurons change their pathways as a result of your experiences and how you think about them, which means mindfulness can be used to overcome negative thought patterns.

The structure of the brain is affected by how you think and tends to form connections that will be revisited if you dwell or brood on a subject and repeatedly think negatively about it, and, in turn, this affects thought patterns. For example, if you tend to think negatively about having to attend a diabetes clinic, because you have to take time off work or wait a long time to be seen, these negative feelings are stored up and rolled out again each time you are invited to attend the clinic.

Negative information and experiences are processed more quickly than positive information and experiences, because as a protective measure the brain registers a negative experience immediately, to prepare us for a quick response at a later date. This has the effect of making us fear similar situations, so we avoid them in future, but these feelings can become internalised, leading to resentment, which can ultimately become depression. In this way, you can create your own stress. However, practising mindfulness – and some advice on how to do that follows – can help reduce stress and enable new neurons to form in the brain, which improves mental clarity.

- By regularly practising mindfulness you can build positive thought pathways about your diabetes self-care and self-management.

- To reduce their hold over you, identify the basis or cause of your negative feelings and emotions. For example, recognise that perhaps you had to wait a long time in the diabetes clinic because they were particularly short-staffed. Try to see the issue from the opposite perspective.

- To practise mindfulness, breathe steadily and deeply while you concentrate fully on the present moment. Focus on the way you are breathing and notice if it is relaxed, loud, easy and so on (it doesn't matter which it is). If your mind wanders, gently bring your attention back to your breathing.

- You can start with just 10 minutes of mindfulness in a session or incorporate mindful awareness into activities such as walking or listening to music. However, it's a good idea to set aside a specific time to practise mindfulness every day.

- The key to successful mindfulness is to regularly acknowledge distractions and regain your focus, while treating your wandering mind with kindness and accepting that distraction is a natural part of the practice.

- There are lots of mindfulness apps, as well as online guided meditation sessions, available.

Improving your emotional health

As we have noted, diabetes tends to be accompanied by changeable emotions, such as depression, which can be treated if recognised and reported (see chapter 4). If you have been feeling low then it's a good idea to see your doctor to find out what help is available. Although it can be hard, talking about how you feel can really help. You may think you are coping well with your diagnosis, but sharing this information with family, friends and work colleagues is very beneficial for you and them.

Being stressed has an adverse effect on your blood glucose levels, especially if this happens often, making it much harder to keep them within healthy limits. Try to be focused about your diabetes by practising mindfulness (see p. 164). If the cause of your stress is a diabetes diagnosis or the onset of complications, this will get easier to cope with as you adapt to the change in your life.

Activity

- At the end of each day, use your behaviour change diary, a notebook, your computer, or phone to reflect on any unhealthy habits that you are aware of, such as depressive eating, because you were bored, fed up, or miserable.

- Write anything down that you think you might have done differently and add what you could have done instead – for example, gone for a walk to lift your mood or phoned a friend and had a laugh to cheer you up. This is a way of cementing new, healthy behaviours into your consciousness.

- Eventually, these healthier behaviours will become second nature and over time this can lead to a number of positive health benefits, as changes occur in the way you think and react to life challenges.

- You could also use your behaviour change diary to record where you have seen successful behaviour changes in others who have similar circumstances to you – for example, someone with type 2 diabetes who walks regularly or who makes a point of talking to others with health issues to gain support.

- Record what you have learned from observing how someone else is trying to achieve their personal goal. Is there anything you can take from this to help you?

- Motivation has been defined as the reason for action. If you lack motivation for diabetes self-care, imagine yourself undertaking an aspect of diabetes self-care and remind yourself why you're doing that task. If you have a strong reason for doing the task you can see yourself achieving it. This is an effective way of bringing an idea into fruition.

Tackling depression

As we have already seen, poor physical health has a negative effect on your psychological health. If depression and anxiety go undiagnosed, this causes an increase in blood glucose levels. It is the case that diabetes can both cause depression, and depression can be a factor in the development of type 2 diabetes. This vicious circle of cause and effect can lead to a reduced quality of life.

Research has shown that taking regular exercise is a natural way to significantly reduce depressive symptoms in people with prediabetes and type 2 diabetes. A reduction in overall blood glucose levels is a key factor in preventing both depression and type 2 diabetes. This suggests that exercise is a significant way to manage depressive symptoms and improve quality of life, especially where the cause of depression is high glucose levels.

It has also been shown that when it comes to depression and type 2 diabetes, some people may feel highly stigmatised by mental illness, deciding that they should be able to cope and 'pull themselves together.' This perception makes them more likely to stop visiting a counsellor or therapist, taking their antidepressants or engaging in self-care activities, which then increases blood glucose levels. However, negativity and the sense that diabetes dictates all the rules can be overcome by:

- **Managing those blood glucose levels:** Remember, elevated glucose levels cause chemical changes in the brain that make depression more likely and more severe if you already have it.

- **Maintaining a regular exercise routine:** This will not only lower your blood glucose levels, it will also lead to the release of 'feel good' hormones (endorphins) that improve your mood and outlook.

- **Not blaming yourself:** If you've done all you can and your prediabetes or type 2 diabetes management is not on target, think positively and congratulate yourself on what you have achieved with your diabetes. As we saw earlier, emotions and feelings have a huge impact on glucose levels and mood, and positivity helps to lift a low mood and lower blood glucose levels.

- **Building resilience:** In relation to diabetes management this describes your capacity to withstand or recover quickly from any difficulties associated with diabetes with a set of management skills and attitudes that can be learned, developed and strengthened over time through intentional practice and effort.

Self-management of prediabetes and type 2 diabetes involves the adoption of positive behaviours and mindfulness to control unhealthy, competing behaviours – for example, going for a walk instead of having a cigarette, or unhealthy snack. This self-control requires self-discipline – you need to recognise the temptation and you need to overcome it – but the satisfaction of having made a good choice will create the necessary motivation to continue that behaviour.

Activity

- Set yourself small, achievable goals to develop positive perceptions of diabetes and improve your sense of mastery over your diabetes self-management. This proactive method is a good way to address any challenges and prevent burnout.

- Recognise that prediabetes or diabetes is only one aspect of your identity.

- Practise activities like smiling and laughing, which can create positive emotional and physical changes, helping to reduce stress and improve your outlook.

- Tell! Whether it's emotional support or help with managing daily diabetes-related tasks, tell friends, family and healthcare providers what you need.

Coping with the unexpected

Rather than simply relying on health professionals, in order to manage diabetes effectively and prevent complications, proactivity and a thorough understanding of the reasons for diabetes self-care and management are crucial. This way of thinking about diabetes self-care encourages the adoption of coping strategies to deal with situations that are not the norm. In turn, this prevents or lessens any stress caused by the changed situation, stopping the brain from expecting difficult situations or events.

If, for example, you are staying with family, it is important to explain to them what your diabetes self-management entails so that they can support you and meet your needs. This means thinking about what you need to take with you so the medicines or foods are available when you need them – never rely on others to provide or pack what you need, unless, of course, you are unable to do this for yourself.

When you're away from home, whether it's for work, you're on holiday or you're going to a party, be mindful of what's going to be on offer and if at all possible make wise choices. If you eat a few party snacks and have a few drinks, for example, recognise that this is not a behaviour you engage in every day and don't let it cause any diabetes anxiety. If you manage your diabetes well and take regular exercise most of the time, your blood glucose levels won't be significantly affected by a slight change to your regular routine.

***RICHARD SAYS:** I used to dread any social event, because of other people's expectations. When I went to my parents' house for Christmas, my mother would keep nagging me to eat, but I felt like she was disrespecting my efforts to manage my blood glucose levels at quite a challenging time of the year. I think she saw my refusal to eat her huge portions and extras as an insult to her hospitality, but my way of coping with this temptation was to have a normal-sized portion and fill up with lots of veg. I had to keep repeating, "I have Type 2 diabetes, Mother!" when the cake, chocolates and mince pies were presented. It's the same with birthdays and any big celebration*

– I just have to stick to my guns and remind myself that I'm looking after myself. I also try to plan ahead and take some of my own lower-carb meals with me. Mum's behaviour has become a bit of a joke now and we tease her, because even the non-diabetic members of the family feel pressured by her.

Several studies have shown that there is a direct link between positive emotional health and lower blood glucose levels in people with (and without) diabetes. Positive emotions help you to cope with stress, leading to reduced stress responses in the body and improved health behaviours that contribute to better glucose control. They also make you more likely to follow health advice – to eat appropriately, exercise regularly and take medication if it's prescribed – and self-manage your diabetes effectively, which in turn means your quality of life is improved and you are likely to live longer. It is a circle, but a virtuous one.

✶ Key messages ✶

- When you receive a diagnosis of prediabetes or type 2 diabetes it is common to wonder how it will change your life, but there is plenty of support available to help you cope with your new situation.

- It is normal to feel stressed, overwhelmed or depressed by your diabetes and the impact of high blood glucose levels on mood contributes to these feelings.

- Taking regular exercise is a natural way to significantly reduce depressive symptoms.

- You can improve your emotional health, diabetes self-management and blood glucose control with techniques that increase your awareness of activities that are unconducive to good health.

- Positive emotional health is strongly associated with positive diabetes self-care behaviours.

A final note

Congratulations on working through the preceding chapters! I hope you've learned a lot about preventing, managing or even reversing prediabetes and type 2 diabetes, and are now well on your way to a diabetes-free life – or at least to improving your blood glucose levels, blood pressure, cholesterol and fitness, not to mention carrying less weight and having more energy!

I have met hundreds of people who have risen to this challenge and made the significant lifestyle changes described in this book. You now have the tools to successfully take control of your lifestyle and your health, so what are you waiting for?

And if you find this book helps you achieve better health, please do tell other people about it, so that they can benefit from it, too.

Good luck! I know you can do it!

Dr Val Wilson

Glossary

Acanthosis nigricans: is the name for velvety areas of skin that usually appear in the armpits, neck or groin.

Acromegaly: a rare condition where the body produces too much growth hormone, causing body tissues and bones to grow more quickly. Over time, this leads to abnormally large hands and feet, and a wide range of other symptoms. Acromegaly is usually diagnosed in adults aged 30–50, but it can affect people of any age.

Adenosine: One of the four nucleoside building blocks of RNA (ribonucleic acid), which are essential for life, adenosine has a controlling effect on the amount of insulin produced by the body and how body cells respond to it.

Adrenocortical hormones: Steroid hormones produced by the outer layer of the adrenal glands located on top of the kidneys. The main adrenocortical hormones are cortisol, which regulates stress, metabolism, and inflammation, and androgens, which contribute to male sex hormone characteristics.

Alzheimer's disease: causes the brain to shrink and brain cells to eventually die. This leads to a gradual decline in memory, thinking, behaviour and social skills. These changes affect a person's ability to function.

Angina pectoris: the medical term for chest pain or discomfort due to coronary heart disease. This occurs when the heart muscle does not receive enough blood because one or more arteries supplying the heart is narrowed or blocked (also called *ischaemia*).

Antioxidant: compounds that scavenge and neutralise free radicals that damage cells and cause illness and ageing.

Antipsychotics: medications prescribed to treat psychosis.

Atherosclerosis: degenerative disease of the arteries associated with fatty deposits on the inner walls, leading to reduced blood flow.

Beta cells: the insulin-producing cells of the pancreas.

Body mass index (BMI): you are classed as overweight if your BMI measures 25–29.9. A BMI of 30–39.9 is classed as obese, while a BMI of 40 or greater is considered to be morbid obesity.

Cataracts: cause a clouding of the lens due to protein deposits, affecting central vision.

Cholecalciferol: also known as vitamin D$_3$, is produced by the skin when exposed to sunlight and is present in certain foods such as dairy products, eggs and fish. Its primary function is to maintain normal calcium and phosphate levels in the serum – the liquid that remains after blood has clotted.

Cholesterol: blood fats.

Colorectal cancer: (sometimes called *colon cancer*) is a disease where cells in the colon or rectum grow out of control. The colon is the large intestine or large bowel. The rectum is the passageway that connects the colon to the anus.

Cortisol: a steroid hormone produced in times of stress that controls mood, motivation and fear.

Cushing's syndrome: a condition where an elevated amount of cortisol hormone is produced over a long period of time. Cortisol helps the body respond to stress, maintaining blood pressure and regulating blood glucose levels.

Dawn phenomenon: sometimes called the dawn effect, this is an observed increase in blood glucose levels that takes place in the early morning, often between 2 a.m. and 8 a.m. This naturally occurring phenomenon is frequently seen among the general population and can affect the management of prediabetes and diabetes.

Dementia: describes the loss of cognitive functioning – thinking, remembering and reasoning – to such an extent that it interferes with a person's daily life and activities. A person with dementia may not be able to control their emotions and their personality may change.

Diastolic blood pressure (bottom number): records the pressure on the vessel walls when the heart is at rest and blood pressure is lowest between beats.

Digital sclerosis: describes tight, thick, waxy skin on your fingers that can cause finger joints to become stiff and hard to move. If blood glucose levels remain high, digital sclerosis can affect other areas of skin and can spread throughout the body.

Dopamine: is a neurotransmitter that allows us to feel pleasure, satisfaction and motivation.

Endorphins: hormones released in response to pain or stress and during pleasurable activities such as exercise, massage, eating and sex. Endorphins help relieve pain, reduce stress and bring a sense of wellbeing.

Epinephrine: norepinephrine promotes the breakdown of triglycerides, a process that enables fat to be utilised as a source of heat. Norepinephrine, also known as adrenaline, is both a neurotransmitter and a hormone. It plays an important role in your body's fight-or-flight response.

Eruptive xanthoma: a skin condition causing benign lesions to appear on the skin that consist of *lipid*, or fatty acid, deposits. They are uncommon and can appear alongside other health conditions. As a result, they may be an early warning sign of another illness that affects the metabolism, such as prediabetes or type 2 diabetes.

Fasting plasma glucose test: measures the amount of glucose in the blood after fasting overnight for 8–12 hours.

Gestational diabetes: develops in around 2–4% of women at around 28 weeks of pregnancy.

Ghrelin: a hormone that stimulates appetite, hunger and promotes fat storage.

Glaucoma: a condition where there is increased pressure within the eyeball, causing gradual loss of sight.

Glucocorticoids: medications prescribed to reduce inflammation. Within the body, glucocorticoids are steroid hormones derived from cholesterol, synthesised and secreted by the adrenal glands.

Gout: an inflammatory arthritis causing pain and swelling in the joints.

HbA1c test: measures the amount of glucose sticking to red blood cells over the 3–4-month lifespan of the cell.

Hyperglycaemia: high blood glucose levels caused by a lack of insulin.

Hypertension: also known as high blood pressure, is a common condition that affects the arteries. Hypertension describes the continually high force of the blood pushing against the artery walls so the heart has to work harder to pump blood.

Hypoglycaemia: is an abnormally low level of glucose in the blood (less than four millimoles per litre). When glucose is very low (below two millimoles per litre), the body doesn't have enough energy to carry out vital functions like respiration, heartbeat and brain activity.

Hypothyroidism: causes many metabolic abnormalities as well as multiple clinical symptoms. Blood glucose may be affected in hypothyroidism and levels can increase. it has been noted that patients with type 1 diabetes who also have hypothyroidism may have higher levels of Haemoglobin A1C (HbA1c).

Impaired fasting glucose: impaired fasting glycaemia (IFG) is another name for prediabetes. Blood glucose levels in the body are raised, but not enough to be type 2 diabetes. IFG means that the body isn't able to use glucose as efficiently as it should.

Impaired glucose tolerance: this term is used when the body is unable to process glucose properly. The diagnosis is made following a blood test showing a raised glucose level confirmed with a glucose tolerance test.

Insomnia: characterised by persistent difficulty falling asleep, staying asleep or getting quality sleep despite having the opportunity to do so.

Insulin resistance: occurs when the cells of the liver, muscles and fat don't respond efficiently to insulin and fail to take up glucose in the blood.

Leptin: a hormone that promotes the burning of fat for energy when carbohydrates are in short supply.

Lipids: a broad range of organic compounds which include fats, waxes, sterols, fat-soluble vitamins such as vitamins A, D, E and K, monoglycerides, diglycerides, phospholipids and others. The functions of lipids include storing energy, signalling and acting as a structural part of cell membranes.

Macrovascular complications: affect the large blood vessels, including the coronary arteries, aorta and large arterioles in the brain and limbs. This results in effects on the body such as high blood pressure, arterial stiffness and kidney disease.

Macular degeneration: leads to a loss of central vision and is usually associated with older age, although hyperglycaemia may trigger onset at an earlier age.

Macular oedema: describes swelling of the macula – the centre of the retina that provides sharp, straight vision – causing blurred or distorted vision.

Maturity onset diabetes (MODY): a type of diabetes that occurs in children which is directly inherited from their parents.

Melatonin: is a hormone produced by the brain in response to darkness. It helps with the timing of your internal clock and sleep patterns.

Metabolic syndrome: a group of associated conditions including obesity, coronary heart disease, high blood pressure, high blood fats (such as cholesterol) and high levels of chemicals that prevent the breakdown of blood clots in the arteries and heart.

Microvascular complications: are long-term complications affecting the small blood vessels. These include retinopathy (affecting the eyes), nephropathy (affecting the kidneys) and neuropathy (affecting the nerves).

Neovascular glaucoma: is the result of high glucose levels damaging the surface of the retina at the back of the eye. This condition causes bleeding, raising eye pressure to encourage new and abnormal blood vessels to grow on the iris (the coloured part of the eye), which increases eye pressure further.

Nephropathy: a condition caused by hyperglycaemia where the nephrons of the kidneys are damaged. Nephropathy causes a persistent and clinically detectable amount of protein in the urine, in association with high blood pressure and reduced kidney function.

Neuropathy: peripheral neuropathy affects the hands, arms and feet, causing pain, numbness, tingling and weakness. Sensory neuropathy results in a loss of sensation in different areas of the body. Autonomic neuropathy affects the function of internal organs such as the bladder, digestive system and heart. Motor neuropathy is a progressive muscle disorder characterised by weakness in different muscles.

Neuroplasticity: where the neurons of the brain are reshaped to form new connections and positive thought patterns.

Non-alcoholic fatty liver disease (NAFLD): a build-up of fat in the liver due to obesity that is linked to insulin resistance.

Norepinephrine: also called noradrenaline, is both a neurotransmitter and a hormone. As a neurotransmitter, it's a chemical messenger that helps transmit nerve signals across nerve endings to another nerve cell, muscle cell, or gland cell.

Oestrogen: is one of the main female sex hormones. It is needed for puberty, the menstrual cycle, pregnancy, bone strength and other functions of the body. Oestrogen levels vary throughout the menstrual cycle and fall after menopause.

Oral glucose tolerance test: measures the rate at which blood glucose rises in response to an amount of glucose taken by mouth.

Ozempic: weight-loss drug. Ozempic is the brand name for semaglutide. Ozempic and Wegovy are not the same, though they contain the same active ingredient, semaglutide.

Pancreatitis: inflammation of the pancreas.

Peripheral vascular disease: is the reduced circulation of blood to a body part other than the brain or heart. It is caused by a narrowed or blocked blood vessel. The main cause is atherosclerosis, which is the build-up of fatty deposits that narrow a blood vessel, usually an artery.

Plaque: describes deposits of low-density lipoproteins on the artery walls, causing narrowing and reducing blood flow.

Polycystic ovary syndrome (PCOS): a condition where the ovaries contain a large number of harmless follicles where eggs develop but cannot be released, so ovulation does not take place.

Prediabetes: describes blood glucose levels that are higher than normal but not high enough to be diagnosed as full-blown type 2 diabetes.

Retinopathy: a chronic eye condition describing a number of symptoms, including abnormal dilation of the blood vessels and bleeds in the retina at the back of the eyes. This can lead to heavy scarring and sight loss.

Sensory polyneuropathy: a common health condition affecting multiple nerves when there is damage due to hyperglycaemia. *Distal polyneuropathy* affects many of the nerves in the hands and feet, leading to reduced ability to feel light touch and lack of awareness of the position of the foot; reduced pain and temperature sensations; tingling and burning sensations; weakness, and sensations like walking on pebbles.

Sleep apnoea: is a relatively common condition where the walls of the throat relax and narrow during sleep, interrupting normal breathing.

Systolic blood pressure (top number): records the pressure on blood vessel walls at its peak as the heart beats.

Transient ischaemic attack (mini-stroke): can cause slurring of speech and/or muscle weakness down one side of the body and may last for a few minutes, hours, or even days.

Triglycerides: a type of fat in the blood that the body uses for energy.

Xanthelasma: yellow growths on or near the eyelids. They can be flat or slightly raised and form when deposits of cholesterol (lipid or fat) build up under the skin. While xanthelasma themselves are not harmful, they can be a sign of high blood glucose levels and cholesterol deposits in blood vessels.

Resources

Websites

Action on Sugar
Action on Sugar is a specialist group concerned with sugar and its effects on health. It aims to work with the food industry and government to provide a consensus on the harmful effects of a high-sugar diet and to bring about a reduction in the amount of sugar in processed foods.
actiononsugar.org

American Diabetes Association
The American Diabetes Association aims to prevent, treat and ultimately cure diabetes on a global scale, and offers support and resources for those with the condition.
diabetes.org

BMI measurement
The NHS has an easy-to-use calculator for working out your BMI measurement.
nhs.uk/live-well/healthy-weight/bmi-calculator

British Heart Foundation
British Heart Foundation funds research into heart and circulatory disease and provides resources to support good health.
bhf.org.uk

Change 4 Life
Change4Life Service is a public health programme in England which began in January 2009, run by Public Health England. It is the country's first national social marketing campaign to tackle the causes of obesity.
nhs.uk/change4life/food-facts/sugar

Combat boredom eating
Boredom eating is a common behaviour, but here are some tips to help you manage it.
hriuk.org/health/nutrition/10-ways-to-combat-boredom-eating

Diabetes UK
Diabetes UK campaigns for better care for those with diabetes and funds research into new treatments.
diabetes.org.uk

Every Body Moves
A website developed by Paralympics UK and Toyota to provide opportunities for everyone to be more active. By entering your post code, the website shows accessible sports available in your area.
everybodymoves.org.uk

Find out your risk of type 2 diabetes
Finding out your risk of type 2 diabetes only takes a few minutes on the Diabetes UK website. Consult your doctor for further advice and help.
diabetes.org.uk/my-risk

Healthier You Diabetes Prevention Programme
The Healthier You NHS Diabetes Prevention Programme, also known as the Healthier You programme, identifies people at risk of developing type 2 diabetes and refers them on to a nine-month, evidence-based lifestyle change programme. If you have any questions about the Healthier You programme, please contact: england.ndpp@nhs.net

How To Reduce Your Child's Sugar Intake
My book for adults and children provides in-depth and achievable ways to cut excess sugar from your life.
London: Robinson, ISBN: 978-1472144898

International Diabetes Federation (IDF)
The IDF is an umbrella organisation of over 250 national diabetes organisations in more than 160 countries or territories. Their mission is to improve the lives of those with diabetes and prevent diabetes in those at risk.
info@idf.org

NHS Digital Weight Management Programme
Available if you are on a waiting list for an operation and have been identified by your hospital as someone who would benefit from participating in the NHS Digital Weight Management Programme.
england.nhs.uk/digital-weight-management/nhs-digital-weight-management-programme

Obesity UK
Obesity UK is a leading charity dedicated to supporting people living with obesity in the UK.
obesityuk.org.uk

Sugar Smart UK
Sugar Smart UK is a campaign run by Sustain to help local authorities, businesses, organisations, workplaces and individuals to reduce the amount of sugar consumed.
sugarsmartuk.org

World Diabetes Foundation
The World Diabetes Foundation is a leading global funder of diabetes prevention and care projects in low-to middle-income countries.
worlddiabetesfoundation.org

World Health Organization Global Diabetes Compact
The WHO Global Diabetes Compact aims to reduce the risk of diabetes, ensuring that all who are diagnosed with diabetes have access to equitable, comprehensive, affordable and quality treatment and care. This work will also support the prevention of type 2 diabetes from obesity, unhealthy diet and physical inactivity.
who.int/initiatives/the-who-global-diabetes-compact

Diabetes cookery books

Cavan, D. and Porter, E. (2018). *The Low-Carb Diabetes Cookbook: 100 Delicious Recipes to Help Control Type 1 and Reverse Type 2 Diabetes*. Vermilion. ISBN-13: 978-1785041402.

Geissler, F. (2024). *Diabetic Diet After 60 for Beginners: Take Care of Your Health With Super Easy and Quick Recipes and a 30-Day Meal Plan for Lasting Diabetes Control*. Independently published. ISBN-13: 979-8343875355.

Goodwin, C. (2025). *Super Easy Diabetic Cookbook for Beginners With Pictures: 2000 Days of Low-Carb and Low-Sugar Recipes to Cook Every Day. The Complete 30-Day Meal Plan to Manage Type 2 Diabetes.* Independently published. ISBN-13: 979-8284925164.

Hairy Bikers. (2020). *The Hairy Bikers Eat to Beat Type 2 Diabetes: 80 Delicious and Filling Recipes to Get Your Health Back on Track* (Foreword by R. Taylor). Seven Dials. ISBN-13: 978-1841884073.

Wellis, P. (2025). *Balanced Diabetic Air-Fryer Cookbook for Beginners: Quick and Healthy Recipes for Type 1 and 2 Diabetes, Newly Diagnosed Prediabetes, and Insulin Resistance. Easy, Low-Carb, Tasty Food With a 30-Day Meal Plan.* Independently published. ISBN-13: 979-8316957279.

Wells, E.O. (2024). *Plant Based Diet Cookbook for Type 2 Diabetes After 40: Delicious Easy-to-Make Plant Based Recipes for Managing Type 2 Diabetes.* Independently published. ISBN-13: 979-8883574565.

References

Introduction

12.1 million adults in the UK were living with either diabetes or prediabetes:

Diabetes UK, 2025: 'One in five adults now live with diabetes or prediabetes in the UK' diabetes.org.uk/about-us/news-and-views/one-five-adults-now-live-diabetes-or-prediabetes-uk

38.4 million adults have type 2 diabetes and 97.6 million have prediabetes:

Centre for Disease Control, 2024: 'National diabetes statistics report' cdc.gov/diabetes/php/data-research/index.html

Only 8% of people with diabetes have type 1:

NICE clinical knowledge summaries, 2025: Diabetes - type 1: How common is it? https://cks.nice.org.uk/topics/diabetes-type-1/background-information/prevalence

1. Exploring definitions of diabetes

A blood glucose level less than 7.8 mmol/L:

Diabetes UK, 2025: 'Diagnostic criteria for diabetes' diabetes.org.uk/for-professionals/improving-care/clinical-recommendations-for-professionals/diagnosis-ongoing-management-monitoring/new_diagnostic_criteria_for_diabetes

A result between 7.8 mmol/L and 11.0 mmol/L:

Diabetes UK, 2025: 'Diagnostic criteria for diabetes' diabetes.org.uk/for-professionals/improving-care/clinical-recommendations-for-professionals/diagnosis-ongoing-management-monitoring/new_diagnostic_criteria_for_diabetes

A reading of more than 11.1 mmol/L:

Diabetes UK, 2025: 'Diagnostic criteria for diabetes' diabetes.org.uk/for-professionals/improving-care/clinical-recommendations-for-professionals/diagnosis-ongoing-management-monitoring/new_diagnostic_criteria_for_diabetes

Losing 5% of your bodyweight:
Diabetes UK, 2025: 'Lose weight' diabetes.org.uk/living-with-diabetes/eating/whats-your-healthy-weight/lose-weight

Type 2, however, makes up 90–95% of cases:
Balk, E.M. et al., 2015: 'Combined diet and physical activity promotion programs to prevent type 2 diabetes among persons at increased risk: a systematic review for the Community Preventative Service Taskforce' *Annals of Internal Medicine* 163: 437–451; Gong, Q.H. et al., 2015: 'Lifestyle interventions for adults with impaired glucose tolerance: a systematic review and meta-analysis of the effects of glycaemic control', *Internal Medicine* 54: 303–310

Type 2 diabetes is usually diagnosed in people who are over 40 years of age:
Diabetes UK, 2025: 'Diagnostic criteria for diabetes' diabetes.org.uk/for-professionals/improving-care/clinical-recommendations-for-professionals/diagnosis-ongoing-management-monitoring/new_diagnostic_criteria_for_diabetes

415 million people globally – or one in 11 of the world's adult population – are living with diabetes:
Diabetes UK, 2023: 'Diabetes prevalence' diabetes.co.uk/diabetes-prevalence.html

Almost half of all global type 2 diabetes cases remain undiagnosed:
Diabetes UK, 2023: 'Diabetes prevalence' diabetes.co.uk/diabetes-prevalence.html

Physical activity, a healthy diet and weight loss can reduce diabetes risk by 58%:
Zaharia, O.P. et al., 2019: 'Risk of diabetes-associated diseases in subgroups of patients with recent onset diabetes: a 5-year follow-up study', *Lancet Diabetes and Endocrinology* thelancet.com/journals/landia/article/PIIS2213-8587(19)30187-1/fulltext

2. Physical symptoms of diabetes

There are nine main day-to-day symptoms:
Medical News Today, 2025: 'What are the early signs of type 2 diabetes?' medicalnewstoday.com/articles/323185

A specific blood test, called an HbA1c test, is usually used:
Diabetes UK, 2025: 'Type 2 diabetes symptoms' diabetes.org.uk/about-diabetes/type-2-diabetes/symptoms

Over the short term – three to five years – only about 25% of people:
Harvard Publishing, 2013: 'Many miss prediabetes wake-up call' health.harvard.edu/blog/many-miss-pre-diabetes-wake-up-call-201303266023

Up to 50% of people with prediabetes can prevent or delay type 2 diabetes:
Diabetes UK, 2025: 'Prediabetes symptoms and risk reduction' diabetes.org.uk/about-diabetes/type-2-diabetes/prediabetes

3. Risk factors you can control

One in 10 adults now risk developing type 2 diabetes by the year 2035:
Diabetes UK, 2021: '1 in 10 adults living with diabetes by 2030' diabetes.org.uk/about-us/news-and-views/1-10-adults-living-diabetes-2030

Walking for 15 minutes after meals could prevent type 2 diabetes:
BBC, 2013: 'Short walks could cut diabetes risk in older people' bbc.co.uk/news/health-22853314#:~:text=Walking%20for%2015%20minutes%20after,-to-moderate%22%20p

Some older people in their seventies or eighties may not be able to produce adequate amounts of insulin:
Muller, D.C., Elahin, D., Tobin, J.D., et al., 1996: 'The effect of age on insulin resistance and secretion: a review', Seminars in Nephrology 16(4): 289–98

13.6 million people are currently at increased risk of developing type 2 diabetes:
BBC, 2016: 'Diabetes: Tenth of adults at risk from disease by 2035' bbc.co.uk/news/health-37720610

Losing weight can reduce this risk by as much as 58%, while regular exercise reduces the risk by 64%:
Francesco, P. et al., 2010: 'Quantity and quality of sleep and incidence of type 2 diabetes' Diabetes Care 33(2): 414–20

Reduce your risk of developing type 2 diabetes:
Centers for Disease Control, 2024: 'Prevent type 2 diabetes: Talking to your patients about lifestyle change' cdc.gov/diabetes/hcp/lifestyle-change-program/index.html#:~:text=58%25%20lower%20incidence%20of%20type,program%20participants%20after%2015%20years

Getting less than six hours' sleep a night:
Diabetes UK, 2025: 'Sleep and diabetes' diabetes.org.uk/guide-to-diabetes/life-with-diabetes/sleep-and-diabetes#:~:text=Risk%20of%20type%202%20diabetes,healthily%20and%20be%20physically%20active

People who smoke are 30–40% more likely to develop type 2:
Centers for Disease Control, 2024: 'How smoking can increase risk for and affect diabetes' fda.gov/tobacco-products/health-effects-tobacco-use/how-smoking-can-increase-risk-and-affect-diabetes#:~:text=Type%202%20Diabetes?-,Does%20Smoking%20Cause%20Diabetes?,

There are 7000 chemicals in one cigarette:
US Department of Health and Human Services, Centers for Disease Control and Prevention, National Center for Chronic Disease Prevention and Health Promotion, Office on Smoking and Health: ncbi.nlm.nih.gov/books/NBK179276/pdf/Bookshelf_NBK179276.pdf#page=592

One in four UK adults currently has metabolic syndrome:
International Diabetes Federation, 2006: 'Metabolic syndrome' idf.org/media/uploads/2023/05/attachments-30.pdf

Three or more of the risk factors I've listed suggests metabolic syndrome:
International Diabetes Federation, 2006: 'Metabolic syndrome' idf.org/media/uploads/2023/05/attachments-30.pdf

Becoming a serious issue in developing countries:
International Diabetes Federation Diabetes Atlas, 2021: 'Global picture' ncbi.nlm.nih.gov/books/NBK581940/#:~:text=As%20explained%20in%20Chapter%202,in%202045%20(Table%203.4)

Due to the increased stress that these factors place on the body:
Wu, Y., Zhang, S., Qian, S.E., et al., 2022: 'Ambient air pollution associated with incidence and dynamic progression of type 2 diabetes: a trajectory analysis of a population-based cohort' BMC Medicine bmcmedicine.biomedcentral.com/articles/10.1186/s12916-022-02573-0#:~:text=Existing%20evidence%20supports%20an%20association,of%20different%20progressions%20of%20T2D

The first research to quantify the contribution of air pollution to disease:
Rao, X., Patel, P., Puett, R. et al., 2015: 'Air pollution as a risk factor for type 2 diabetes', The Society of Toxicology, Oxford University Press

4. Risk factors you can't control

One in nine adults has prediabetes:

Diabetes UK, 2025: 'Diabetes risk factors' cdc.gov/diabetes/communication-resources/prediabetes-statistics.html

There are six key risk factors:

Diabetes UK, 2025: 'Diabetes risk factors' diabetes.org.uk/about-diabetes/type-2-diabetes/diabetes-risk-factors#:~:text=Your%20risk%20increases%20with%20age,Diabetes%20information%20in%20other%20languages

Medicines such as *glucocorticoids*, *antipsychotics* and some HIV treatments:

Diabetes UK, 2025: 'Diabetes risk factors' diabetes.org.uk/about-diabetes/type-2-diabetes/diabetes-risk-factors#:~:text=Your%20risk%20increases%20with%20age,Diabetes%20information%20in%20other%20languages

Hormonal conditions such as *Cushing's syndrome*:

Diabetes UK, 2025: 'Diabetes risk factors' diabetes.org.uk/about-diabetes/type-2-diabetes/diabetes-risk-factors#:~:text=Your%20risk%20increases%20with%20age,Diabetes%20information%20in%20other%20languages

Sleep disruption due to conditions such as *sleep apnoea*:

Diabetes UK, 2025: 'Diabetes risk factors' diabetes.org.uk/about-diabetes/type-2-diabetes/diabetes-risk-factors#:~:text=Your%20risk%20increases%20with%20age,Diabetes%20information%20in%20other%20languages

When Tom was diagnosed in 2013:

Diabetes Australia, 2013: 'Tom Hanks type 2 diabetes diagnosis' diabetesaustralia.com.au/blog/tom-hanks-type-2

After the age of 35, the risk of developing prediabetes and subsequently type 2 diabetes increases:

Diabetes UK, 2025: 'Diabetes risk factors' diabetes.org.uk/about-diabetes/type-2-diabetes/diabetes-risk-factors#:~:text=Your%20risk%20increases%20with%20age,Diabetes%20information%20in%20other%20languages

Those who develop prediabetes and type 2 diabetes before the age of 40:

Diabetes UK, 2025: 'Diabetes risk factors' diabetes.org.uk/about-diabetes/type-2-diabetes/diabetes-risk-factors#:~:text=Your%20risk%20increases%20with%20age,Diabetes%20information%20in%20other%20languages

Men aged 35 to 54 years are twice as likely to develop type 2:
Diabetes UK, 2025: 'Diabetes risk factors' diabetes.org.uk/about-diabetes/type-2-diabetes/diabetes-risk-factors#:~:text=Your%20risk%20increases%20with%20age,Diabetes%20information%20in%20other%20languages

Rates of type 2 diabetes have risen four times faster in men aged 35 to 54:
Nursing Times, 2009: 'Men at greater risk of diabetes' nursingtimes.net/primary-care/men-at-greater-risk-of-diabetes-13-07-2009/#:~:text='Most%20of%20them%20will%20have,'

Type 2 tends to develop later in women:
PMC, 2025: 'Type 2 diabetes in women' pmc.ncbi.nlm.nih.gov/articles/PMC10716945/

If you are from an Afro-Caribbean, Black African or South Asian (Indian, Pakistani, Bangladeshi) background:
Diabetes UK, 2025: 'Diabetes and ethnicity' diabetes.org.uk/about-diabetes/type-2-diabetes/diabetes-ethnicity#:~:text=Age%20and%20ethnicity,could%20help%20lower%20your%20risk

More common in younger people from a South Asian background:
Diabetes UK, 2025: 'Diabetes and ethnicity' diabetes.org.uk/about-diabetes/type-2-diabetes/diabetes-ethnicity#:~:text=Age%20and%20ethnicity,could%20help%20lower%20your%20risk

The level of risk is as follows:
Diabetes UK, 2025: 'Diabetes risk factors' diabetes.org.uk/about-diabetes/type-2-diabetes/diabetes-risk-factors#:~:text=You're%20two%20to%20six%20times%20more%20likely,if%20you've%20ever%20had%20high%20blood%20pressure

There are a number of medical conditions associated:
Diabetes UK, 2025: 'Related conditions' diabetes.org.uk/about-diabetes/looking-after-diabetes/related-conditions#:~:text=If%20you%20have%20type%202,depression

AI could also detect who is at risk of type 2 diabetes 70% of the time:
BBC, 2024: 'Hospitals trial AI to spot type 2 diabetes risk' bbc.co.uk/news/articles/c80v1p5l4n1o

5. Chronic complications

Eight serious complications of undiagnosed or long-term high blood glucose levels:
NHS, 2025: 'Type 2 diabetes complications' nhs.uk/conditions/type-2-diabetes/complications/#:~:text=damage%20to%20

your%20blood%20vessels,gum%20disease; Diabetes UK, 2025: 'Complications' diabetes.org.uk/about-diabetes/looking-after-diabetes/complications

72% of people have already developed significant problems:
International Diabetes Federation, 2023: 'More than two in three people with diabetes already have complications at diagnosis' idf.org/news/more-than-two-in-three-people-with-diabetes-already-have-complications-at-diagnosis; CDC, 2024: 'Lifestyle change program' cdc.gov/diabetes/hcp/lifestyle-change-program/index.html

Normalise blood glucose levels and prevent 90% of eye disease:
National Eye Institute, 2019: 'Diabetes and vision loss prevention' nei.nih.gov/sites/default/files/2019-06/diabetes-prevent-vision-loss.pdf

In those over 40 years of age and in people who smoke:
Diabetes & Metabolic Syndrome Journal, 2019: 'Public health policies and programs' dmsjournal.biomedcentral.com/articles/10.1186/s13098-019-0482-2#:~:text=Public%20health%20policies%20and%20programs,most%20clinical%20guidelines%20%5B21%5D

7.4 million people in the UK currently living with heart and circulatory problems:
MedicAlert, 2025: 'Heart condition statistics' medicalert.org.uk/heart-condition/#:~:text=Currently%2C%20there%20are%20around%20 7.4,are%20held%20in%20member%20records

Mark Labbett – the Beast on UK TV quiz *The Chase*:
Wales Online, 2021: 'The Chase star Mark Labbett diagnosed with diabetes during a routine check-up' walesonline.co.uk/lifestyle/tv/chase-star-mark-labbett-diagnosed-21057188

6. Mindset changes

Eating something with a lot of fat and/or sugar:
HealthXchange, 2025: 'Why we crave high-fat, high-sugar foods' healthxchange.sg/food-nutrition/food-tips/why-crave-high-fat-high-sugar-foods#:~:text=High%2Dsugar%20and%20 high%2Dfat%20foods%20not%20only%20taste,serotonin)%20 which%20give%20us%20feelings%20of%20pleasure

Sugar ... which can then become addictive:
HealthXchange, 2025: 'Why we crave high-fat, high-sugar foods' healthxchange.sg/food-nutrition/food-tips/why-crave-high-fat-high-sugar-foods#:~:text=High%2Dsugar%20and%20

high%2Dfat%20foods%20not%20only%20taste,serotonin)%20 which%20give%20us%20feelings%20of%20pleasure; PMC, 2008: 'Sugar addiction' pmc.ncbi.nlm.nih.gov/articles/PMC2235907

The same endorphin hit is true of exercise:
Healthline, 2025: 'How to increase endorphins' healthline.com/health/how-to-increase-endorphins

Intensive in-person or online diabetes education course:
Diabetes UK, 2025: 'Type 2 diabetes and me' diabetes.org.uk/guide-to-diabetes/managing-your-diabetes/education/type-2-diabetes-and-me

Be prescribed glucose-lowering medication:
NHS, 2025: 'Type 2 diabetes treatment' nhs.uk/conditions/type-2-diabetes/treatment/#:~:text=Medicine%20for%20type%202%20diabetes,or%20having%20a%20%22hypo%22

Dopamine levels can be increased by reducing saturated fat intake:
Nutritionist Resource, 2025: 'Dopamine: How what we eat impacts our brain chemistry' nutritionist-resource.org.uk/articles/dopamine-how-what-we-eat-impacts-our-brain-chemistry#:~:text=Foods%20high%20in%20saturated%20fat,lack%20of%20motivation%20and%20drive

For six weeks, it is likely that you will be in the right mindset:
Mentalzon, 2025: '66 days to build a new habit – why it's not a myth but real habit psychology' mentalzon.com/en/post/7770/66-days-to-build-a-new-habit-why-it%E2%80%99s-not-a-myth-but-real-habit-psychology#:~:text=Where%20the%20Number%2066%20Came,average%2C%20not%20a%20magic%20deadline

Nine months to become something you automatically do:
The Conversation, 2025: 'Forming new habits can take longer than you think – here are 8 tips to help you stick with them' theconversation.com/forming-new-habits-can-take-longer-than-you-think-here-are-8-tips-to-help-you-stick-with-them-255118#:~:text=How%20long%20does%20it%20really,is%2C%20and%20who's%20doing%20it

It takes, on average, 66 days to change a habit:
University College London, 2009: 'How long does it take to form a habit?' ucl.ac.uk/news/2009/aug/how-long-does-it-take-form-habit#:~:text=4%20August%202009,the%20behaviour%20is%20performed%20automatically

7. Physical changes

Many physical and emotional benefits to carrying less body fat:
HealthTalk, 2025: 'Mental and emotional benefits of losing weight' healthtalk.org/experiences/weight-change-associated-health-problems/mental-and-emotional-benefits-losing-weight

Contributes to around 70% of weight-loss success:
Nutrition.org.uk, 2025: 'Obesity, healthy weight loss and nutrition' nutrition.org.uk/health-conditions/obesity-healthy-weight-loss-and-nutrition

Exercise accounts for the remaining 30%:
Vox, 2018: 'Exercise and weight loss myth' vox.com/2018/1/3/16845438/exercise-weight-loss-myth-burn-calories

Losing 5% of your bodyweight:
Diabetes UK, 2025: 'Lose weight' diabetes.org.uk/living-with-diabetes/eating/whats-your-healthy-weight/lose-weight

A BMI measurement of above 25 increases your risk of type 2 diabetes:
NHS, 2025: 'Obesity' nhs.uk/conditions/obesity/#:~:text=The%20psychological%20problems%20associated%20with,in%20blood%20pressure%20during%20pregnancy

Meal replacement milkshakes contain a great deal of sugar (some up to 50%):
Healthline, 2025: 'Meal replacement shakes' healthline.com/nutrition/meal-replacement-shakes#:~:text=Some%20Contain%20Unhealthy%20Ingredients,a%20few%20grams%20of%20sugar

30–70% of people have no access to weight management services local to them:
NICE, 2025: 'Draft guidance' nice.org.uk/guidance/the14/documents/draft-guidance#:~:text=for%20this%20guidance.-,Unmet%20need,commitments%20or%20me

Demand for it to help weight loss has outstripped research:
IQVIA, 2025: 'Outlook for obesity in 2025' qvia.com/locations/emea/blogs/2025/01/outlook-for-obesity-in-2025-more-than-a-transition-year

Resulting in a 15% loss in bodyweight (20% with the drug Mounjaro):
MedsRus, 2025: 'Uropa vs Mounjaro' medsrus.co.uk/blog/uropa%20-vs-mounjaro#:~:text=Efficacy%20in%20Weight%20Loss,believed%20to%20enhance%20this%20effect

'Sudden death' attributed to the diabetes drug itself:
Motley Rice, 2025: 'Diabetes lawsuits' motleyrice.com/diabetes-lawsuits/uropa/safe-for-weight-loss/deaths

Caused by damage to the optic nerve:
European Medicines Agency, 2025: 'PRAC concludes eye condition NAION very rare side effect of semaglutide medicines' ema.europa.eu/en/news/prac-concludes-eye-condition-naion-very-rare-side-effect-semaglutide-medicines-ozempic-rybelsus-wegovy#:~:text=EMA's%20safety%20committee%20(PRAC)%20has,taking%20semaglutide%20for%20one%20year

Losing between 5 and 7% of your bodyweight:
Mayo Clinic, 2025: 'Diabetes prevention' mayoclinic.org/diseases-conditions/type-2-diabetes/in-depth/diabetes-prevention/art-20047639#:~:text=The%20American%20Diabetes%20Association%20recommends,almost%2060%25%20over%20three%20years

Losing weight reduces the risk of developing prediabetes by 58%:
Mayo Clinic, 2025: 'Diabetes prevention' mayoclinic.org/diseases-conditions/type-2-diabetes/in-depth/diabetes-prevention/art-20047639

Sticking to this regime to prevent type 2 diabetes from returning:
NHS, 2024: 'Third of NHS "soups and shakes" participants in remission from type 2 diabetes in a year' england.nhs.uk/2024/08/third-of-nhs-soups-and-shakes-participants-in-remission-from-type-2-diabetes-in-a-year/#:~:text=News-,Third%20of%20NHS%20%E2%80%9Csoups%20and%20shakes%E2%80%9D%20participants%20in%20remission%20from,over%2010kg%20in%20one%20year

Steak, sausages, ham and bacon could increase the risk:
University of Cambridge, 2024: 'Red and processed meat consumption associated with higher type 2 diabetes risk' mrc-epid.cam.ac.uk/blog/2024/08/21/red-processed-meat-type-2-diabetes-risk-interconnect

Calcium supplementation reduced fasting plasma insulin:
PubMed, 2019: 'Calcium and insulin' pubmed.ncbi.nlm.nih.gov/31071733/#:~:text=Meta%2Danalyses%20were%20carried%20out,multiple%20dosing%20schedules%20are%20needed

Associated with elevated blood glucose (hyperglycaemia) and insulin resistance:
Barbagallo, M. and Dominguez, L.J., 2015: 'Magnesium and type 2 diabetes' pmc.ncbi.nlm.nih.gov/articles/PMC4549665

Waist circumference is independently associated with low magnesium levels:
PMC, 2023: pmc.ncbi.nlm.nih.gov/articles/PMC9844104

lowers blood glucose and, in turn, prevents or reverses prediabetes:
PMC, 2023: pmc.ncbi.nlm.nih.gov/articles/PMC9844104

Lower post-meal levels of glucose:
PMC, 2012: pmc.ncbi.nlm.nih.gov/articles/PMC3254006

Vitamin D supplements can help reduce obesity, BMI and waist circumference:
Frontiers in Nutrition, 2025: 'Vitamin D and obesity' frontiersin.org/journals/nutrition/articles/10.3389/fnut.2025.1664960/full

These activities are associated with a 20-30% risk reduction:
PubMed, 2008: pubmed.ncbi.nlm.nih.gov/18071167

Increased physical activity is especially beneficial for weight reduction:
PMC, 2014: pmc.ncbi.nlm.nih.gov/articles/PMC3925973/#:~:text=The%20rationale%20for%20exercise%20within,always%20encourage%20an%20active%20lifestyle

Brisk walking at a moderate intensity per week reduces diabetes risk by 27%:
BMJ Group, 2025: bmjgroup.com/faster-walking-speed-of-4-km-hour-linked-to-significantly-lower-type-2-diabetes-risk

Regular exercise reduces the risk of developing type 2 diabetes by 40%:
John Pounds Centre, 2025: johnpoundscentre.co.uk/blog/regular-exercise-cuts-diabetes-risk-by-up-to-40-per-cent#:~:text=Regular%20exercise%20cuts%20diabetes%20risk,conducted%20jointly%20with%20Cambridge%20University

Reduce the risk of heart disease and stroke:
NHS, 2025: nhs.uk/conditions/coronary-heart-disease/prevention/#:~:text=You%20should%20also%20try%20to,Give%20up%20smoking

Acts to reverse prediabetes in the same way as treating prediabetes:
NHS, 2025: nhs.uk/conditions/type-2-diabetes/treatment/#:~:text=Lifestyle%20changes%20to%20help%20with,Don't

Ongoing beneficial effect on glucose levels that can last up to 24 hours:
University College London, 2024: 'Exercise boosts memory 24 hours after workout' ucl.ac.uk/news/2024/dec/commentary-exercise-boosts-memory-24-hours-after-workout-new-research

Children and teenagers are now eating three times more sugar:
Diabetes Research & Wellness Foundation, 2025: drwf.org.uk/news-and-events/news/warning-over-young-people-s-sugar-intake-as-study-finds-children-could-be-three-times-over-the-recommended-daily-amount

Twice the maximum recommended level of sugar per day:
Diabetes Research & Wellness Foundation, 2025: drwf.org.uk/news-and-events/news/warning-over-young-people-s-sugar-intake-as-study-finds-children-could-be-three-times-over-the-recommended-daily-amount

The recommended level of daily fibre is 30g for adults:
NHS, 2025: nhs.uk/live-well/eat-well/digestive-health/how-to-get-more-fibre-into-your-diet

Average diet contains only one-fifth starchy carbohydrates:
NHS, 2015: 'Starchy foods and carbohydrates' nhs.uk/live-well/eat-well/food-types/starchy-foods-and-carbohydrates/#:~:text=Starchy%20foods%20%E2%80%93%20such%20as%20potatoes,skin%20on%20for%20more%20fibre

Adults in the UK only consume an average of 19g of fibre daily:
Diabetes UK, 2025: 'Fibre and diabetes' diabetes.org.uk/living-with-diabetes/eating/carbohydrates-and-diabetes/fibre-and-diabetes

Dietary fibre for those aged 16 years and upwards is 30g:
Diabetes UK, 2025: 'Fibre and diabetes' diabetes.org.uk/living-with-diabetes/eating/carbohydrates-and-diabetes/fibre-and-diabetes

Only 9% achieve this:
NHS, 2025: nhs.uk/live-well/eat-well/digestive-health/how-to-get-more-fibre-into-your-diet

Dark (not milk) chocolate a week is linked to a 21% reduced risk:
British Medical Journal, 2024: 'Eating dark but not milk chocolate linked with reduced risk of type 2 diabetes' bmjgroup.com/eating-dark-but-not-milk-chocolate-linked-to-reduced-risk-of-type-2-diabetes

A 2014 study found that intermittent fasting improved prediabetes:
Diabetes UK, 2025: 'Intermittent fasting for remission' diabetes.org.uk/about-diabetes/type-2-diabetes/remission/intermittent-fasting-for-remission

Increase your metabolic rate by over 3.6%:
PMC, 2018: pmc.ncbi.nlm.nih.gov/articles/PMC5783752

Raspberries contain tannin and a substance that blocks the breakdown of starch:
Healthline, 2025: 'Raspberry nutrition' healthline.com/nutrition/raspberry-nutrition

Eating 500ml of frozen raspberries reduces triglyceride blood fats:
Healthline, 2025: 'Raspberry nutrition' healthline.com/nutrition/raspberry-nutrition

There is a link between stress-induced anxiety and depression:
Mayo Clinic, 2025: 'Depression and anxiety' mayoclinic.org/diseases-conditions/depression/expert-answers/depression-and-anxiety/faq-20057989

Stress can indirectly increase the risk of type 2 diabetes:
PMC, 2022: pmc.ncbi.nlm.nih.gov/articles/PMC9561544

Stored glucose is released by the liver to provide energy for 'the fight':
NCBI Bookshelf, 2025: ncbi.nlm.nih.gov/books/NBK560599

Insulin, which doesn't work well alongside the stress hormone, cortisol:
Veri, 2025: veri.co/learn/cortisol-insulin-resistance?srsltid=AfmBOorlkDqUsPGSkwfP5ZYjUzMl1ycApkndbjuxugmnqpQyx6fzrBSj

Cortisol encourages stored glucose to be released from the liver:
Levels, 2025: levels.com/blog/guide_to_cortisol

Blood glucose level was 8% higher than on days when they didn't have caffeine:
Lane, J. (2004). 'Caffeine Impairs Glucose Metabolism in Type 2 Diabetes'. *Diabetes Care* 27(8):2047–2048

Two cups of percolated coffee or four cups of black tea per day:
Lane, J. (2004). 'Caffeine Impairs Glucose Metabolism in Type 2 Diabetes'. *Diabetes Care* 27(8):2047–2048

Decaffeinated coffee also increased blood glucose levels:
Diabetes Journals, 2014: 'Caffeinated and Decaffeinated Coffee Consumption' diabetesjournals.org/care/article/37/2/569/29536/Caffeinated-and-Decaffeinated-Coffee-Consumption

Reduces insulin sensitivity by affecting the processes that use or store glucose:
PubMed, 2001: pubmed.ncbi.nlm.nih.gov/11575527

Significant association between prediabetes and chronic pain symptoms:
PMC, 2020: pmc.ncbi.nlm.nih.gov/articles/PMC7333061

People with prediabetes are also at increased risk of *sensory polyneuropathy*:
PMC, 2017: pmc.ncbi.nlm.nih.gov/articles/PMC5583955

Enhancing peripheral nerve regeneration in the hands and feet:
PMC, 2017: pmc.ncbi.nlm.nih.gov/articles/PMC5583955

Lowering systolic blood pressure by 5 mmHg:
The Lancet, 2021: thelancet.com/journals/lancet/article/PIIS0140-6736(21)01920-6/fulltext

Can reduce the risk of type 2 diabetes by as much as 16%:
The Lancet, 2021: thelancet.com/journals/lancet/article/PIIS0140-6736(21)01920-6/fulltext

The levels of 184 different fat molecules in the blood can help to predict:
New Scientist, 2025: newscientist.com/article/2310609-fat-levels-in-blood-predict-risk-of-type-2-diabetes-and-heart-disease

High levels of HDL cholesterol can lower:
Heart UK, 2025: heartuk.org.uk/genetic-conditions/high-hdl-cholesterol

And the higher the number of daily cigarettes, the greater the risk:
Diabetes Research & Wellness Foundation, 2025: drwf.org.uk/news-and-events/news/smoking-linked-with-higher-risk-of-type-2-diabetes

Smokers are 30–40% more likely to develop type 2 diabetes than non-smokers:
Diabetes Research & Wellness Foundation, 2025: drwf.org.uk/news-and-events/news/smoking-linked-with-higher-risk-of-type-2-diabetes

850,000 people currently live with undiagnosed prediabetes and type 2:
East Basildon PCN, 2025: eastbasildonpcn.nhs.uk/news/diabetes-awareness

13.6 million people are at risk from these conditions:
Notts ICB, 2025: notts.icb.nhs.uk/preventing-type-2-diabetes

Reduces the risk of developing type 2 diabetes by up to 40%:
University College London, 2016: 'Regular exercise can cut your diabetes risk' ucl.ac.uk/news/2016/oct/some-good-more-better-regular-exercise-can-cut-your-diabetes-risk

5 mmHg has been shown to reduce the risk of developing type 2 diabetes:
The Lancet, 2021: thelancet.com/journals/lancet/article/PIIS0140-6736(21)01920-6/fulltext

8. Emotional health

Sustained stress can lead to inflammatory changes:
PMC, 2017: pmc.ncbi.nlm.nih.gov/articles/PMC5476783

Common in those with long-term elevated glucose levels:
CVRTI, University of Utah, 2025: cvrti.utah.edu/the-role-of-inflammation-in-diabetes-related-heart-complications

Negative emotions also impact the immune response:
New Scientist, 2025: newscientist.com/article/dn4116-brain-study-links-negative-emotions-and-lowered-immunity

Positive about your health releases feel-good hormones:
Harvard Health, 2025: health.harvard.edu/mind-and-mood/feel-good-hormones-how-they-affect-your-mind-mood-and-body

Bad energy is physically reflected:
WebMD, 2025: webmd.com/balance/signs-negative-energy

Poor emotional health can worsen diabetes management:
PMC, 2024: pmc.ncbi.nlm.nih.gov/articles/PMC11979121

Sharp glucose fluctuations that directly affect mood:
University of Michigan School of Public Health, 2019: sph.umich.edu/pursuit/2019posts/mood-blood-sugar-kujawski.html

In 2018, Public Health England did some research:
Public Health England, 2018: Health matters: Preventing Type 2 Diabetes gov.uk/government/publications/health-matters-preventing-type-2-diabetes

You will undertake around 95% of your diabetes care yourself:
Making Diabetes Easier, 2025: makingdiabeteseasier.com/uk/managing-diabetes/target-blood-glucose-levels; PubMed, 2021: pubmed.ncbi.nlm.nih.gov/33797970

Diabetes burnout can lead people to ignore their diabetes:
Diabetes UK, 2025: diabetes.org.uk/living-with-diabetes/emotional-wellbeing/diabetes-burnout; Patient.info, 2025: patient.info/features/diabetes/what-you-should-know-about-diabetes-burnout; BSW Health, 2025: bswhealth.com/blog/diabetes-distress-coping-with-the-emotional-toll-of-diabetes

Psychologically speaking, it is normal for people:
Oxford Academic, 2025: academic.oup.com/jcem/article/110/Supplement_2/S131/8042169; Diabetes UK, 2025: diabetes.org.uk/living-with-diabetes/emotional-wellbeing/depression; Diabetes UK, 2025: diabetes.org.uk/living-with-diabetes/emotional-wellbeing/diabetes-burnout

Emotional health tends to rise the longer you've had the condition:
PMC, 2025: pmc.ncbi.nlm.nih.gov/articles/PMC12264664

In turn, this affects thought patterns:
MDPI, 2025: mdpi.com/2227-9032/12/14/1457

Negative information and experiences are processed more quickly:
Lucidity, 2025: lucidity.org.uk/negativity-bias-why-we-remember-negatives-more-acutely

The brain registers a negative experience immediately:
Verywell Mind, 2025: verywellmind.com/negative-bias-4589618

Diabetes can both cause depression:
Diabetes UK, 2025: diabetes.org.uk/living-with-diabetes/emotional-wellbeing/depression#:~:text=Depression%20and%20diabetes-,Depression%20and%20diabetes,a%20factor%20in%20developing%20it; PMC, 2016: pmc.ncbi.nlm.nih.gov/articles/PMC4863499

Depression can be a factor in the development of type 2 diabetes:
Diabetes UK, 2025: diabetes.org.uk/about-us/news-and-views/depression-risk-factor-type-2-diabetes-our-research-reveals; PubMed, 2006: pubmed.ncbi.nlm.nih.gov/16520921; *DMS Journal*, 2024: dmsjournal.biomedcentral.com/articles/10.1186/s13098-024-01273-4; *Guardian*, 2023: theguardian.com/society/2023/sep/07/depression-can-play-direct-role-in-developing-type-2-diabetes-says-study

Exercise is a natural way to significantly reduce depressive symptoms:
Harvard Health, 2025: health.harvard.edu/mind-and-mood/exercise-is-an-all-natural-treatment-to-fight-depression; Mental Health Foundation, 2025: mentalhealth.org.uk/explore-mental-health/publications/how-improve-your-mental-health-using-physical-activity; PMC, 2024: pmc.ncbi.nlm.nih.gov/articles/PMC11298280

People may feel highly stigmatised by mental illness:
American Psychiatric Association, 2025: psychiatry.org/patients-families/stigma-and-discrimination#:~:text=Public%20stigma%20involves%20the%20negative,relative%20to%20other%20health%20care; psychiatry.org/patients-families/stigma-and-discrimination; Mind, 2025: mind.org.uk/news-campaigns/news/half-of-uk-adults-believe-there-is-still-a-great-deal-of-shame-associated-with-mental-health-conditions

Direct link between positive emotional health and lower blood glucose:
PMC, 2025: pmc.ncbi.nlm.nih.gov/articles/PMC12474718

Acknowledgements

I've enjoyed working with Holly Jarrald and Caroline Hewlett at Bloomsbury and without their editing expertise and guidance this book would not have been possible. I'd also like to thank all the generous people from my 'diabetes database' who allowed me to use their anonymous personal stories to help others trying to prevent, improve or reverse their prediabetes and type 2 diabetes. My biggest debt of all, though, is to my husband for his constant patience, support, useful suggestions, the loan of his laptop to complete this book when mine suddenly died, and for the very flattering author photo!

Index

acanthosis nigricans   70
acromegaly   51
addiction to sugar   75, 125, 126, 128
adrenocortical hormone   125
age factors, prediabetes and type 2 diabetes   19, 28, 41, 42–3, 54
alcohol consumption   32, 75, 76, 113, 134–5, 145–6
allergies/intolerances, food   106
alpha-lipoic acid   114
Alzheimer's disease   32
angina pectoris   63–4
ankles, swollen   60
antipsychotic medications   41, 49, 136
appetite suppression   107–10
arteries, narrowing   33, 64–6, 145
arthritis   128, 141, 156
atherosclerosis   36, 64, 66, 69, 71
autonomic neuropathy   62, 63

behaviour, changing   74–6, 153–4
   beginning the process of change   75–8
   breaking a habit   76, 91–5
   coping strategies   85, 90
   embracing the challenge   93
   keeping a behaviour change diary   76–8, 83, 85, 87, 91, 107, 121, 142, 147, 165–6
   overcoming barriers to change   77, 85, 91–5
   stage 1 – precontemplation of change   79–80
   stage 2 – contemplation of change   81–3
   stage 3 – planning a change   83–6
   stage 4 – action   86–8
   stage 5 – maintenance   90–1
   support for   86, 87, 88, 89, 92, 94, 95
   what to do if you relapse   91–5
   see also lifestyle changes
berberine   114–15
bipolar disorder and risk of prediabetes and type 2 diabetes   49
bladder infections   61
blame, self-   156, 158, 167
blind spots   56, 57, 61
blood clots   33, 34, 64
blood fats *see* cholesterol (blood fats)
blood glucose meters   142
blood pressure   36–8, 41, 49, 64, 114–15, 136, 142–4, 147
   lowering   142–3, 147, 154
blurred vision   22, 43, 57–8
body fat/fat storage   30, 34, 41, 45, 49, 117–18, 128, 131, 143, 147
body mass index (BMI)   99–100

boredom, eating out of 92–3
brain function 32, 125, 163–4
British Medical Journal 132

caffeine and blood glucose
    levels 23, 32, 140–1
calcium and insulin function 115
calorie requirements weight loss,
    adult 111
cancer medication and blood
    glucose levels 136
cancer risks 98, 101, 110, 113,
    130, 146, 149, 156
carbohydrates 19, 58, 122–4
  fibre 112, 122–3, 124, 129
  glycaemic index (GI)
    values 130–2
  starches 124, 129
  sugars 38, 75, 106, 123,
    124–7, 129, 145, 146
cardiac arrhythmia 63
cataracts 58, 59
celebrating successes 85, 88,
    90, 95
chest pain and tightness 56, 60,
    63–4, 65
Chinese medicine 114–15
chlorella and blood glucose
    levels 115
chocolate, dark 132
cholesterol (blood fats) 34, 64,
    136, 143, 144–6, 147
  high-density lipoproteins
    (HDL cholesterol) 34, 145
  low-density lipoproteins
    (LDL cholesterol) 34,
    145, 146
  and smoking 145–6, 147–8
  triglycerides 34, 145, 146

chromium and insulin
    resistance 115
chronic complications, recognising
    and dealing with 56–71
cinnamon, health benefits of 115
circulatory problems 22, 33, 56,
    65–6, 147
cold hands and feet 56, 57, 64,
    65, 66, 67, 151
comfort eating 75, 76, 105, 107,
    134–5
complex (healthy)
    carbohydrates 122–3
corticosteroids and blood glucose
    levels 136
cortisol (stress hormone) 49, 51,
    125, 128, 134, 135
Cushing's syndrome 41, 51
cuts, scratches and bruises, slow
    healing 21, 22, 56–7, 65,
    67, 156

darkening skin 23, 70
dehydration 22, 24, 138–40
dementia risk 32
dental issues 57, 68–9, 152, 153
depression and anxiety 32, 50–1,
    134, 162–3, 165, 166–7, 169
diabetes *see* type 1 diabetes;
    type 2 diabetes
diabetes education courses 82
diarrhoea 61, 63
diary, keeping a behaviour
    change 76–8, 83, 85, 87,
    91, 107, 121, 142, 147, 165–6
diastolic blood pressure 37
diet and dieting
  commercial weight-loss
    plans 103–4

common setbacks   105-6
emotional consequences of   104-5
healthy food choices   92, 101, 112-13, 122, 124, 147, 154
meal timing   132-3
NHS diabetes reversal programme   111
planning and goal setting   83-6
portion sizes   86, 87, 90-1, 103
processed foods   109, 112-13, 124, 126, 130, 131
see also carbohydrates; weight loss
dietary fibre   112, 122-3, 124, 129, 146
digital sclerosis   70
dizziness/light-headedness   37-8, 61, 139
DNA   46-7
doctors/professional medical support
   advice and help with lifestyle changes   82, 83, 84, 86, 92, 104, 106, 118, 120, 145
   diabetes medication   42, 82-3, 102, 106-10, 122, 137, 138, 169
   and emotional health   50, 159-60
   help quitting smoking   92, 147, 149-50
   importance of keeping appointments   150-3
   managing high blood pressure and cholesterol issues   143, 144, 146, 147
   pre-existing medical conditions   49-53

   recognising and dealing with chronic complications   56-71
   reporting your symptoms   21, 24, 32, 36, 49-53
   testing for prediabetes and type 2 diabetes   19, 24, 25, 28, 42, 102, 106
   see also dental issues; opticians and ophthalmologists
dopamine levels   75, 92

emotional health   155-6
   behaviour change diary   165-6
   coping with changes to routine, e.g. social events   168-9
   depression and anxiety   32, 50-1, 134, 162-3, 165, 166-7, 169
   'diabetes burnout'   162
   exercise/physical activity   166, 167, 169
   improving   162-9
   mindfulness and stress management   162-4
   responding to diagnosis   156-61
   stress and blood glucose levels   17, 43, 49, 134-5, 141, 165, 166, 169
   tackling depression   165-6
endorphins   75, 167
energy drinks   23
environmental factors and risk of prediabetes and type 2 diabetes   38, 47
epinephrine and exercise   120
erectile dysfunction   44, 57, 61, 69-70
eruptive xanthoma   70

ethnicity and risks of prediabetes and type 2 diabetes   41, 42, 44–5, 54
exercise and physical activity   18, 20, 29–31, 116–21, 122, 135, 141–2, 143, 147, 154, 166–7, 169
eyesight/eye diseases   18, 22, 27, 44, 56, 57–9, 71, 153

fast-food and obesity   126
fasting plasma glucose test   17, 24, 25
fatigue *see* tiredness
fats, unhealthy   71, 92, 101, 106, 113, 132, 145, 146
  see also cholesterol (blood fats)
fibre, dietary   112, 122–3, 124, 129, 146
fish oil supplements   115
floaters, eye   57
food allergies/intolerances   106
food diary, keeping a   85
  see also diary, keeping a behaviour change
food labels
  fat content   146
  sugar content   106, 126, 127, 128
foot problems   56–7, 67–8
  see also cold hands and feet
fruit and fructose   112, 125, 127–8, 130–1, 133

gender influence of prediabetes and type 2 diabetes risk   41, 43–4, 54
genetics   41, 46–8
genitals, itching   22

gestational diabetes   46, 52–3
ghrelin and appetite/fat storage   125
ginseng and cell death   136
glaucoma   58–9
glucocorticoids   41
glucose intolerance, sleep and   31
glucose tolerance tests   25
glycaemic index (GI) values   130–2
goal setting   84–6, 94, 147, 167
gout   128
growth hormone   49, 51
gum disease   57, 68–9

habits, breaking/changing   76, 91–5
hair loss, lower body   70
Hanks, Tom   42
HbA1c test   17, 24, 25, 28
headaches   32, 43, 60, 129, 139
healthy eating *see* diet and dieting
heart attacks   36, 37–8, 64, 71, 144
heart/cardiovascular disease   33, 34, 36, 41, 42, 44, 49, 56, 63–5, 69, 71, 113, 126, 128, 143, 145, 147
high blood pressure   36–8, 41, 49, 64, 136
  lowering   142–3, 147, 154
high intensity exercise   120
HIV treatments and insulin resistance   41
hormonal changes and conditions, risk of prediabetes and type 2 diabetes   41, 51–2
hypertension (high blood pressure) *see* high blood pressure
hypothyroidism   49, 136

infections and blood glucose
    levels   70, 138
inflammation   112, 125, 141,
    155-6
insomnia   32
insulin-enabling nutrients
    114-16
insulin, prescribed   19, 108, 142
insulin resistance   10, 19-20,
    115-16
  and caffeine   140
  cholesterol levels   144, 147
  ethnicity   44-5
  and fat   30, 34, 117, 147
  and healthy foods   130, 133
  and hormones   41, 49, 51
  inflammation and chronic
    pain   141
  medications   41, 137, 143
  metabolic syndrome   34-5, 144
  nicotine/smoking   33, 34, 51,
    147, 149
  personal medical history
    49-52
  sleep disturbance   31, 32, 41
  and stress   141
intermittent fasting   132-3
irritability   60, 158
itchiness   22, 70

kidney disease (nephropathy)   18,
    27, 44, 60, 113
kidney function, reduced   56,
    59-61, 71, 144

Labbett, Mark   67
labels, food see food labels
lactose   125, 130-1
leptin   125

levothyroxine and blood glucose
    levels   136
libido (sex drive)   57
life expectancy   42
lifestyle changes   153-4
  exercise   27, 29-31
  sleep   31-2
  smoking   33-4
  weight loss   27, 29-31
  see also behaviour, changing;
    diet and dieting; exercise and
    physical activity
light halos   57
limbic system   125
liver disease (NAFLD),
    non-alcoholic fatty   41, 49
liver function   11, 134, 147
losing weight
  see diet and dieting; exercise;
    weight loss
low-carbohydrate diets   52, 125
  see also carbohydrates; diet and
    dieting
low-fat diets
  see diet and dieting
low intensity exercise   118

macrovascular blood
    pressure   143
macular degeneration
    (macular oedema)   58
magnesium, health benefits
    of   115
maturity onset diabetes
    (MODY)   46
meal replacements   103, 104
meal sizes   86, 87, 90-1, 103
meal timing   132-3
meats, processed   112-13

medical appointments, keeping 150-3
medication
  blood pressure 136, 143
  cholesterol control 146
  and increased risk of prediabetes and type 2 diabetes 11-12, 41, 49, 136-7
  treatment of diabetes 42, 82-3, 102, 107-10, 122, 137, 138, 169
melatonin and insulin function 31
menopause 51-2
mental health 49-51
  see emotional health; stress and blood glucose levels
metabolic syndrome 34-5, 141, 143, 144
metformin 48, 102, 137, 138
microvascular blood vessels 143
mindfulness 163-4
mindset change see behaviour, changing
mini strokes 65-6
moderate intensity exercise 118, 120, 154
motivation for change, your 83, 84, 86
motor neuropathy 62
Mounjaro see weight-loss drugs
muscle mass 44, 100, 109, 110

nausea 60, 61
negative though patterns 163-4
neovascular glaucoma 58-9
nephrons 60, 71
nerve damage (neuropathy) 18, 23, 56, 61-3, 66, 141-2

neurons 32, 163
neuropathy (nerve damage) see nerve damage (neuropathy)
neuroplasticity 163
nicotine see smoking; vaping
non-alcoholic fatty liver disease (NAFLD) 41, 49
non-diabetic hyperglycaemia 25
norepinephrine and energy levels 120
numbness and tingling in legs, hands and feet 23, 56, 57, 61, 66, 67-8, 151, 152

obesity 30, 34, 39, 101, 126, 141, 143, 154
octreotide and insulin production 136
opticians and ophthalmologists 57, 59, 152, 153
oral diazoxide and blood glucose levels 136
oral glucose tolerance test 17, 24, 24
organ rejection medication and blood glucose levels 136
oestrogen 51, 52, 125
Ozempic (Semaglutide/Wegovy) 107-10

pain and blood glucose levels 141-2
pain response, reduced 56, 61, 141
pancreas 10, 11, 16, 20, 42, 54, 109, 136
pedometers 118-19
peripheral neuropathy 62, 63, 141
peripheral vascular disease 66

physical activity *see* exercise and physical activity
plaque
   arterial   64, 69, 145
   dental   68-9
pollution and prediabetes and type 2 diabetes risk   38
polycystic ovary syndrome (PCOS)   41, 49
portion sizes, meal   86, 87, 90-1, 103
positivity and blood glucose levels   169
potassium levels   116
potato carbohydrate content   128
prediabetes   10, 11, 12, 20, 17, 141
   controllable risk factors   27-39
   diagnosis   17-18, 24, 25, 156-61
   fixed risk factors   40-54
   medical appointments   17-18, 24, 25, 150-2
   risk of type 2 diabetes   27-8, 29, 42-3, 96-7
   symptoms overview   21-3
   see also diet and dieting; doctors/professional medical support; exercise and physical activity; weight loss
prednisone and insulin production   136
pregnancy *see* gestational diabetes
processed foods   109, 112-13, 124, 126, 130, 131
   see also refined processed carbohydrates (white carbs)
psychosis medication   41, 49, 136

raspberries, benefits of eating   133
refined processed carbohydrates (white carbs)   19, 35, 58, 98, 112, 114, 123, 130, 131-2
resilience, building personal   167
resistance exercise   120
retinopathy   58, 110
rewarding yourself   85, 88, 90, 95
risk factor overview   26-9, 42
   age   41, 42-3, 54
   blood pressure   36-8
   environmental   38-9
   ethnicity   41, 42, 44-5, 54
   fixed   40-1
   gender   43-4, 54
   genetics   46-8
   gestational diabetes   52-3
   hormonal conditions   51
   medical history   49-53
   mental health   49-51
   metabolic syndrome   34-5
   sleep quality   31-2
   smoking   33-4, 39
   weight and physical activity levels   29-31, 39
   see also individual risks by name

St John's Wort, blood glucose levels and   137
salt intake and blood pressure   113
salt reduction   38, 113, 143, 146
saturated fats   71, 92, 101, 106, 132, 146
schizophrenia and the risk of prediabetes and type 2 diabetes   49

self-blame   156, 158, 167
sensory neuropathy   62
sensory polyneuropathy   141
sexual problems   44, 57, 61, 69–70
sight problems *see* eyesight/eye diseases
silent heart attack   36, 37–8
skin complaints,
   acanthosis nigricans   70
   darkening   23, 70
   eruptive xanthoma   71
   itching   22, 70
   skin tags   23
   slow healing   21, 22, 56–7, 65, 67–8, 156
   thickening   67, 68, 70
   xanthelasma   71
   yeast infections/thrush   22, 70
sleep   31–2, 42, 135
   apnoea   41
SMART goals, setting   94
smoking   33–4, 39, 51, 62, 75, 76, 97, 134–5, 145–6, 147–50, 154
social events, dealing with   168–9
stair climbing as exercise   120
starches/starchy carbohydrates   124, 129
statins and blood glucose levels   52, 136
stress and blood glucose levels   17, 43, 49, 134–5, 141, 165, 166, 169
stroke risk   28, 33, 41, 42, 49, 66, 113, 143, 144, 145, 147
sucrose   123, 131
sugar and sugar consumption   38, 75, 85, 101, 106, 123, 124–7, 129, 145, 146

supplements, dietary   114–15, 136–7
support, getting social   86, 87, 88, 89, 92, 94, 95, 165, 167
swollen ankles   60
symptoms overview, prediabetes and type 2 diabetes   21–3
   see also chronic complications, recognising and dealing with; individual symptoms by name
systolic blood pressure   37, 143, 154

temperatures, reduced response to   56, 61
TENS machines   63
testing for prediabetes and type 2 diabetes   17, 24, 25, 28
thiazide and blood glucose levels   137
thirst   21, 22, 24, 32, 43, 138–40
thrush/yeast infections   22, 70
thyroid dysfunction   49, 136
tingling and numbness in legs, hands and feet *see* numbness and tingling in legs, hands and feet
tiredness   21, 22, 23, 24, 32, 43, 60, 64
trans-fats   146
transient ischaemic attacks (mini strokes)   65–6
triglycerides   34, 145, 146
type 1 diabetes   11, 18
type 2 diabetes   10, 11, 12, 18–19, 20
   controllable risk factors   27–39
   diagnosis   19, 24, 25, 28, 48, 156–61
   fixed risk factors   41–54

chronic complications,
   recognising and dealing
   with   56–71
 symptoms overview   21–3
 see also diet and dieting;
   doctors/ professional medical
   support; exercise and
   physical activity; weight loss

uric acid levels   128
urinate, need to   21, 22, 24, 32,
   44, 59, 60
urine colour   59–60

vaginal dryness   57
vaping   33, 149–50
   see also smoking
vascular disease   66
vigorous sustained exercise   118
visceral fat   10, 45, 117, 147
   see also waist measurement
vision, blurred   22, 43, 57–8
vitamin B3 and blood glucose
   levels   137
vitamin C and D and blood glucose
   levels   116

waist measurement   30, 34,
   45, 49
 healthy adult
   measurements   100
 and risk of prediabetes and type
   2 diabetes   41
walking as exercise   27, 118–20
weakness, limb   61, 154
weight loss   18, 20, 27, 111
 benefits of   111
 commercial weight-loss
   plans   103–4
 due to high blood glucose
   levels   22
 lowering blood pressure   143
 understanding BMI   99–100
 see also behaviour, changing;
   diet and dieting; exercise and
   physical activity
weight-loss drugs   107–10, 154
weight management courses
   106

xanthelasma   71

yeast infections   22, 70